THE COMPLETE IDIOT'S GUIDE® TO

Eating Well with IBS

by Kate Scarlata, R.D., L.D.N.

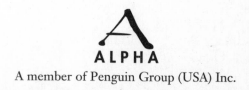

ALPHA

A member of Penguin Group (USA) Inc.

ALPHA BOOKS

Published by the Penguin Group

Penguin Group (USA) Inc., 375 Hudson Street, New York, New York 10014, USA

Penguin Group (Canada), 90 Eglinton Avenue East, Suite 700, Toronto, Ontario M4P 2Y3, Canada (a division of Pearson Penguin Canada Inc.)

Penguin Books Ltd., 80 Strand, London WC2R 0RL, England

Penguin Ireland, 25 St. Stephen's Green, Dublin 2, Ireland (a division of Penguin Books Ltd.)

Penguin Group (Australia), 250 Camberwell Road, Camberwell, Victoria 3124, Australia (a division of Pearson Australia Group Pty. Ltd.)

Penguin Books India Pvt. Ltd., 11 Community Centre, Panchsheel Park, New Delhi—110 017, India

Penguin Group (NZ), 67 Apollo Drive, Rosedale, North Shore, Auckland 1311, New Zealand (a division of Pearson New Zealand Ltd.)

Penguin Books (South Africa) (Pty.) Ltd., 24 Sturdee Avenue, Rosebank, Johannesburg 2196, South Africa

Penguin Books Ltd., Registered Offices: 80 Strand, London WC2R 0RL, England

Copyright © 2010 by Kate Scarlata, R.D., L.D.N.

International Standard Book Number: 978-1-61564-029-4
Library of Congress Catalog Card Number: 2009943485

12   11   10   8   7   6   5   4   3   2   1

Interpretation of the printing code: The rightmost number of the first series of numbers is the year of the book's printing; the rightmost number of the second series of numbers is the number of the book's printing. For example, a printing code of 10-1 shows that the first printing occurred in 2010.

Printed in the United States of America

Note: This publication contains the opinions and ideas of its author. It is intended to provide helpful and informative material on the subject matter covered. It is sold with the understanding that the author and publisher are not engaged in rendering professional services in the book. If the reader requires personal assistance or advice, a competent professional should be consulted.

The author and publisher specifically disclaim any responsibility for any liability, loss, or risk, personal or otherwise, which is incurred as a consequence, directly or indirectly, of the use and application of any of the contents of this book.

Most Alpha books are available at special quantity discounts for bulk purchases for sales promotions, premiums, fund-raising, or educational use. Special books, or book excerpts, can also be created to fit specific needs.

For details, write: Special Markets, Alpha Books, 375 Hudson Street, New York, NY 10014.

Publisher: *Marie Butler-Knight*
Associate Publisher/Acquiring Editor: *Mike Sanders*
Senior Managing Editor: *Billy Fields*
Senior Development Editor: *Christy Wagner*
Senior Production Editor: *Megan Douglass*

Cover Designer: *Rebecca Batchelor*
Book Designer: *Trina Wurst*
Indexer: *Angie Bess*
Layout: *Ayanna Lacey*
Proofreader: *John Etchison*

Contents at a Glance

Contents

18 Perfect Pasta and Pizza   217

19 Eat Your Veggies!   231

Appendixes

Introduction

Are you frustrated with your troubling IBS symptoms? Feel like anything new you eat will trigger an upset? But tired of the same old bland foods you know are "safe"?

It's time to take back your life, take control, and feel your best. As an IBS sufferer, I understand how you feel and appreciate the bumpy road you likely have been traveling. Uncovering the role of your diet and its relationship to how you feel is key to living your best life with IBS.

If you're tired of feeling bloated all the time, constantly racing to the bathroom, or hoping to be more regular, this book is for you. Once you connect the dots from your diet to your personal symptoms, you can begin to make the necessary changes and embark on your new and improved IBS-managed life.

Many factors can contribute to your IBS spinning out of control. In this book, you learn how your lifestyle, digestion process, and food choices impact how you feel. And with the tips to make small changes with big results provided in the following pages, you'll soon be living the life you want, with fewer and fewer IBS outbreaks.

How to Use This Book

This book is divided into three parts:

Part 1, "A Closer Look at IBS and Its Triggers," provides all you need to know about your IBS body and how it is different. You'll gain an understanding of how diet can trigger IBS and when to follow up with your doctor for particularly unruly IBS symptoms. You also learn to manage your lifestyle choices to maximize digestion and minimize your IBS symptoms.

Part 2, "Smart Strategies for IBS-Free Living," launches you right into the grocery store with tips for creating the smartest grocery cart in town. Strategies for keeping food portions "just right" for your IBS body and knowing how to get exactly what you need at your favorite restaurant are also included. I also provide a guide on how to pack all the essentials needed when traveling to keep your traveling tummy happy.

Part 3, "Recipes for Eating Well with IBS" includes all the best-tasting recipes your IBS body can handle—160 of them! Great recipes for your best breakfast favorites, fruit and yogurt smoothies, tasty snacks, satisfying soups, sandwiches, salads, and veggie side dishes. Of course, I also give you plenty of savory entrées. And to make this section complete, I give you two chapters on desserts!

Extras

In every chapter, I've scattered some boxes filled with fun facts, nutritional information, and helpful tips. Be on the lookout for these:

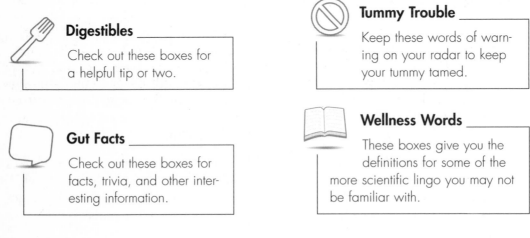

Digestibles

Check out these boxes for a helpful tip or two.

Tummy Trouble

Keep these words of warning on your radar to keep your tummy tamed.

Gut Facts

Check out these boxes for facts, trivia, and other interesting information.

Wellness Words

These boxes give you the definitions for some of the more scientific lingo you may not be familiar with.

Acknowledgments

A big thank you to everyone who helped make this book possible, most notably my husband, Russell, for picking up my slack at home and keeping me laughing! You are the most creative person I know! A special thank you to my three children, Chelsea, Kevin, and Brennan, for understanding my long hours on the computer and for taste-testing all my recipes! Thanks to my extended family and friends for their support. Many thanks especially to my good friends, Liz Oteri and Meg Joyce, for sharing their culinary skills and preparing some fabulous soup recipes for me! Thanks to Sara Caton, for having my back and providing positive commentary!

Thanks to Marilyn Allen, my fabulous agent, and Margaret Furtado for making our introduction. Thanks to Patsy Catsos, for sharing her recipes and nutrition expertise. Thanks to Mike Sanders and Christy Wagner for their editorial expertise. A big thanks to all the researchers "down under" at Monash University in Australia and their continued research in the area of FODMAPs and IBS.

Special Thanks to the Technical Reviewer

The Complete Idiot's Guide to Eating Well with IBS was reviewed by an expert who double-checked the accuracy of what you'll learn here, to help us ensure that this book gives you everything you need to know about eating well with IBS. Special thanks are extended to Sophia Kamveris, M.S., R.D., L.D.

Sophia is a registered dietitian and fellow IBS sufferer who maintains a private practice in the greater Boston area, specializing in nutritional health and wellness counseling. She can be reached at www.sophiakamveris.com.

Trademarks

All terms mentioned in this book that are known to be or are suspected of being trademarks or service marks have been appropriately capitalized. Alpha Books and Penguin Group (USA) Inc. cannot attest to the accuracy of this information. Use of a term in this book should not be regarded as affecting the validity of any trademark or service mark.

Part 1

A Closer Look at IBS and Its Triggers

Understanding what's happening in your IBS body helps you appreciate why certain foods can cause your symptoms. Because IBS varies from one person to another, it's not always easy to decipher what sets your body in a tailspin. In Part 1, you learn about the role of diet in your IBS body and discover what you need to fine-tune to avoid IBS flare-ups.

Part 1 also details how foods are properly absorbed in the body and how to maximize your digestion. You learn about food allergies versus food intolerances and their relationship to IBS. Probiotics are reviewed, introducing the most recent research. With just a few adjustments to your diet and lifestyle, you'll feel better than you have in a long time!

Chapter 1

Living Well with an IBS Diagnosis

In This Chapter

- A look at just what IBS is
- Types of IBS
- How your IBS body is different
- Your diet and symptoms
- Is it more than IBS?

Living with sensitive intestines is just a day in the life for the person with irritable bowel syndrome (IBS). Although experts do not know what causes IBS, certain conditions contribute to its overall picture. IBS is not a one-size-fits-all diagnosis, as symptoms vary from one person to another. Because your IBS body reacts personally to your food intake, learning how to adjust your diet specifically for you is important.

In this chapter, you learn what makes your IBS body function differently, the role of diet triggers, and when you should seek further medical intervention. You gain an insight into the types of IBS and where you fit in.

Most notably, you begin to become part of the solution in getting your life back and effectively managing your IBS.

What Is IBS, Anyway?

IBS, or irritable bowel syndrome, is a collection of symptoms that occur in your digestive tract when nerves and muscles don't work correctly. Here are some common symptoms of IBS:

- Cramping
- Abdominal pain
- Diarrhea
- Gas
- Bloating

- Constipation
- Mucus in the stool
- Changes in bowel habits
- Sense of an incomplete bowel movement

IBS is a chronic condition with no known cure. It's considered a diagnosis of exclusion, as it's often diagnosed when all other conditions or diseases have been ruled out. It's also called a functional gut disorder because there are no visual abnormalities or abnormal medical tests that indicate the intestine is not functional, yet there remains disorder in how the nerves and muscles function in the digestive tract. Many treatments can make you feel better, including diet modifications, as well as physician-recommended medications such as laxatives, antispasmodics, and antidepressants. Some alternative therapies, such as enteric-coated peppermint oil pills, can improve symptoms because peppermint leaves contain oils that relax intestinal muscles and provide pain relief.

Stress does not cause IBS, but I bet you know it can aggravate your symptoms. Helpful stress-management strategies include counseling, therapy, and hypnosis. In fact, a recent study review revealed that 80 percent of those with IBS who tried hypnosis reported symptom relief.

Different Types of IBS

IBS typically falls into three primary categories:

- Constipation-predominant
- Diarrhea-predominant
- A combination of the two

For the constipation-predominant IBS sufferer, increasing fiber can be helpful. Keeping the bowels moving and minimizing constipation is key. This can be done with dietary changes such as increasing the amount of fiber-rich foods you eat. If diet isn't enough, over-the-counter (OTC) fiber supplements can be helpful. Try psyllium husk or methylcellulose, which are soluble fiber–based supplements. Soluble fiber is the better-tolerated form of fiber for IBS. (Read more on fiber basics for IBS in Chapter 2.)

For the diarrhea-predominant IBS sufferer, adding soluble fiber may improve stool formation by adding bulk to it. Soluble fiber forms a gel in the intestines and can help absorb some of the extra fluids causing diarrhea. Tolerance to fiber varies from person to person.

Treatment options for the different types of IBS are often based on whether your symptoms are mild, moderate, or more severe. For this reason, it's very important that you discuss your symptoms, their severity, and their impact on your life as clearly and accurately as possible with your doctor. Together you can work toward managing your IBS as effectively as possible.

 Tummy Trouble

For some with IBS, adding fiber to the diet can make the situation worse. Fiber works for some, but not for everyone. Remember, eating well with IBS requires a personal approach.

What Makes Your IBS Body Different?

With IBS nerve and muscle malfunctions occurring in the intestine, this impacts the way they move in your body and how you interpret the resulting pain. Experts have found that those with IBS have a combination of the following:

◆ Intestinal motility disorder, which occurs when abnormal movement of the intestines is either too fast or too slow, contributing to diarrhea or constipation.

◆ Visceral hypersensitivity, which means your intestines are more sensitive to pain.

◆ Increased levels of serotonin, a chemical found in the gastrointestinal tract. Normally, serotonin is moved out of the intestine, but this is not the case in IBS. This contributes to exaggerated pain sensation.

You may experience some symptoms more or less severely depending on how your body is affected by these factors. Although IBS comes in various shapes and forms, the most universal component is bloating, as 92 percent of IBS sufferers share this symptom.

A bad gastrointestinal "bug" or infection can lead to IBS, and this is called post-infection IBS. We also know that hormones during the premenstrual cycle can act as an intestinal relaxant and can bring on IBS symptoms.

In many cases, you can blame your aunt, mother, and/or granddaddy because IBS runs in families. Researchers have found that your risk for IBS doubles if you have a family member with IBS.

You see, IBS comes in all shapes, sizes, and forms!

You Are Not Alone

IBS is a fairly common condition, affecting 15 to 20 percent of the world's population and is found most commonly in women. IBS generally begins before the age of 35.

Many with IBS do not seek help from a physician and suffer in silence. I know this firsthand, as I've uncovered many patients who have IBS but were too embarrassed to speak about their condition with their doctor.

Your doctor relies on your input in making an assessment of your health status. Being an active advocate for yourself helps your doctor treat you more successfully.

Be Part of the Solution

Don't be afraid to discuss how you feel or what you've been experiencing with a medical professional. Believe me, there's nothing you could say to a doctor that they've not heard before.

Getting proper medical care, whether from your primary care doctor or a gastro-enterologist, a doctor who specializes in digestive issues, is an important step in managing your IBS. Be sure to include a registered dietitian (R.D.) who specializes in IBS in your treatment plan as well.

Digestibles

Finding a R.D. to work with you can be a great asset. Call the American Dietetic Association at 1-800-877-1600 or visit eatright.org to find a R.D. near you.

The Diet–IBS Connection

Uncovering diet culprits in IBS can be tricky. Sometimes it's not what you ate, but how much you ate, and under what conditions. For instance, if you are stressed when eating, that could set you off. If you ate too much ice cream, such as three large scoops versus one small scoop, the portion, not the food choice, could be to blame.

Certainly some foods are common triggers, and you'll learn all about them in the pages to come. But there are many reasons why what you eat seems to send you over the edge.

Your Eating Style

Your best eating style with IBS should allow for frequent small meals consumed in a relaxed atmosphere. Grazing is good for your digestion. Be sure to take your time chewing food thoroughly to kick-start the digestion process. Prepare meals you enjoy eating. Never, ever allow yourself to get overhungry, because being famished leads to grabbing foods on the run, usually unhealthy food choices, setting you up for a bellyache.

If you feel rushed in the morning, set your alarm clock 15 minutes earlier—that's what I do! Bring snacks with you, too, to avoid getting hungry while you're away from home. (More on eating habits and your digestion lifestyle in Chapter 5.)

What's Malabsorption?

One of the main functions of the small intestine is to absorb nutrients from the foods we eat. Malabsorption occurs when something interferes with this process. Malabsorbed foods often contribute to symptoms of IBS. Food that's not absorbed properly makes its way to the large intestine, where the bacteria that reside there get busy fermenting it. While they work, the bacteria produce gas. For many with IBS, fermentable carbohydrates can be a problem. (I know *fermentable carbohydrates* may sound like a term you'd hear in a science lab or winery, but in a way, your body is similar to a science lab!)

Wellness Words

Malabsorption occurs when your body has difficulty absorbing nutrients from food. **Fermentable carbohydrates** (also known as fermentable sugars) are dietary sugars your body can't fully digest and absorb.

You'll learn all about these troublemakers in Chapter 2. Any food that's not absorbed, such as the fermentable carbohydrates, can irritate your large intestine. Carbohydrates that are malabsorbed occur for a number of reasons, including ...

- Lack of digestive enzymes, such as in lactose intolerance.

- Motility disorders that cause the intestine to contract abnormally, interfering with adequate absorption.

- Intestinal wall damage, which can occur due to a virus.

- Inflammation.

- Surgical removal of part of the small intestine.

Not all carbohydrates are troublesome for the person with IBS. You'll soon learn which carbohydrates work best for your IBS body.

When IBS Is Unmanageable

If dietary, medical, and other health-care measures don't offer any relief, you might have something else, or something else in addition to IBS. A number of disorders such as celiac disease, bacterial overgrowth, food allergies, or unusual food intolerances may warrant further investigation.

Work with your physician, gastroenterologist, or registered dietitian to explore less-common conditions you might be experiencing. Never assume you need to continue to feel terrible.

Red Flag Symptoms

Physicians evaluating your symptoms will often run you through a battery of tests to be sure nothing serious is causing your digestive complaints. Having been there, I can tell you that these tests are not always a walk in the park. But they are important because IBS can mimic more serious diseases. These tests are part of the IBS diagnostic process.

Some red flag symptoms your physician will evaluate include the following:

- Anemia
- Gastrointestinal bleeding
- Unexplained weight loss
- Night sweats

- Recent antibiotic use

- Fever

- Thyroid dysfunction

- Osteoporosis or osteopenia

- Family history of colorectal cancer, inflammatory bowel disease, or celiac disease

Irritable bowel is not a disorder you should self-diagnose. IBS shares some warning signs with more concerning health problems such as ovarian and colon cancer. Fortunately, those with IBS are at no greater risk to develop cancer of the intestines, but do be sure you've been adequately screened for more serious health problems if you or your doctor feels this is warranted.

Ruling Out Disorders

Common underlying disorders such as lactose intolerance can complicate IBS management. Other less commonly known issues such as fructose malabsorption, *small intestinal bacterial overgrowth* (SIBO), and delayed food sensitivities may also be present.

Small intestinal bacterial overgrowth is another condition linked with IBS. SIBO occurs when large numbers of bacteria, normally found in the large intestine, take residence in the small intestine. This imbalance can contribute to more severe IBS symptoms. Treatment of SIBO includes antibiotic therapy.

Wellness Words

Small intestinal bacterial **overgrowth** (SIBO) occurs when the small bowel is overrun with bacteria not normally found there.

Work closely with your doctor to uncover all the potential contributors to what's irritating your bowel. IBS management is truly in its infancy, and although great strides have been made to manage symptoms, the scientific community remains mystified in some challenging cases. I know, because I had a difficult IBS case. But with perseverance and good doctors, I was able to learn how to manage my symptoms, which has greatly affected my quality of life.

If your IBS is unruly, don't accept the status quo. Learn all you can to best manage your IBS symptoms and get back your best life. You're on your way just by taking the positive step of reading this book … good job!

The Least You Need to Know

◆ IBS comes in diarrhea-predominant, constipation-predominant, and a combination of both.

◆ Treatment for IBS may involve diet, medications, and stress management.

◆ Be an active part of your own medical team. Don't be passive in your intestinal health.

◆ Food allergies, intolerances, and other conditions can make IBS more difficult to manage.

◆ Small intestine bacterial overgrowth is a treatable condition that mimics IBS and can make symptoms more severe.

Chapter 2

Carbohydrates: Fermentable Sugars and Fiber

In This Chapter

- Meet lactose and fructose
- Your adequate calcium and vitamin D needs
- FODMAPs and your IBS symptoms
- Fiber and the IBS connection

You've got to eat, but sometimes finding the right foods to keep your body happy can be a challenge. IBS comes in all shapes and sizes, and discovering your personal triggers may require a bit of detective work on your part. Understanding the impact of certain foods on your body helps you appreciate why minimizing or eliminating them makes you feel your best. And yes, you deserve to feel great!

In this chapter, we look at carbohydrates, uncovering those that are particularly problematic in IBS. You may have heard about lactose and maybe even fructose, but maybe you haven't heard of some of the others. In this chapter, we take a closer look at these troublemakers and begin to adjust your diet on your way to eating well with IBS.

Lactose Intolerance

Got milk? Or maybe not! *Lactose*, the sugar found in milk and dairy products, can be a menace for those with IBS. Consuming lactose-containing products can lead to gas, bloating, and diarrhea often within 30 minutes and up to 2 hours after indulging in these foods. Many of us lack the digestive enzyme *lactase*, which breaks lactose into two simple forms of sugar, glucose and galactose, so it can be properly absorbed in the small intestine. When you have a deficiency of this enzyme, you can become *lactose intolerant*.

Wellness Words

Lactose is a milk sugar found in milk and dairy foods. **Lactase** is the digestive enzyme needed to digest lactose. **Lactose intolerance** is the inability to digest lactose due to the lack of lactase. **Osmotic diarrhea,** or watery diarrhea, occurs when water is pulled into the intestines when foods aren't properly digested.

When undigested lactose travels into your colon, also known as the large intestine, it's met by millions of intestinal bacteria (we all have these), which ferment the lactose and produce hydrogen or methane gas. These millions of bacteria, estimated at weighing 2 pounds or more, enjoy a feast, and the end product of their party is bloating and a lot of pain for you. And if that's not bad enough, the undigested sugar also sets off a reaction that often results in watery diarrhea. Can it get any better? This type of diarrhea is called *osmotic diarrhea* and occurs when your body draws excess water into the intestine almost in an attempt to dilute the undigested food.

Know Your Threshold

It's estimated that 60 percent of adults are lactose intolerant, or cannot digest the sugar in milk. In fact, most mammals lose the ability to digest lactose after the weaning stage in infancy. Asians and African Americans are more prone to lactose intolerance. People of Northern European descent are more likely to retain their ability to digest lactose, revealing a genetic component.

Even in those with lactose intolerance, some lactose in the diet doesn't pose any problem. Many people have a threshold of lactose absorption, allowing for some digestion. Learning your threshold is an important part of minimizing your IBS symptoms.

Studies have shown that many with lactose intolerance can tolerate up to 1 or 2 cups of milk per day, a range of 11 to 22 grams of lactose. Yet the threshold for lactose varies widely, and for some, a chocolate candy bar that contains just 2 grams of lactose can lead to trouble. (See the "Lactose Content of Common Foods" table later in this chapter for lactose amounts in common foods.)

Lactose Sources

Lactose content in food varies widely, and milk, evaporated milk, and dry milk products provide the largest amounts. Soft cheeses such as ricotta and cottage cheese contain less than milk but still ample lactose. On the other hand, hard cheeses such as Parmesan and cheddar cheese have very little to no lactose.

Gut Facts _____

Milk chocolate candy has some lactose, while dark chocolates vary but often have none.

Hidden lactose can be found in frozen waffles, pancakes, breakfast cereals, margarine, candy, salad dressings, even seasoned potato chips. Some medications have added lactose, too. If you're troubled by the tiniest amount of lactose, be aware of concealed dairy sources that may indicate lactose is present, such as these:

- Butter
- Cheese
- Cream
- Curds

- Dry milk solids
- Milk by-products
- Whey

As you can see in the following table, milk and ice cream are big lactose sources, while hard cheeses and butter have minimal amounts.

Lactose Content of Common Foods

Food	Serving Size	Lactose
Milk	1 cup	11 grams
Ice cream	½ cup	6 grams
Yogurt	1 cup	5 grams
Cottage cheese	½ cup	2 or 3 grams
American cheese	⅓ cup	2 grams

continues

Lactose Content of Common Foods   (continued)

Food	Serving Size	Lactose
Butter	2 tablespoon	trace amounts
Cheddar cheese	⅓ cup	0 grams
Parmesan cheese	1 tablespoon	0 grams

Meeting Your Calcium and Vitamin D Needs

If you omit dairy products from your diet to avoid the problems associated with lactose intolerance, you not only decrease the dairy foods, you also decrease your calcium and vitamin D sources.

Calcium provides structure to your body's skeleton, so this mineral is essential for bone health. But there's more: calcium is necessary for muscle contraction, nerve transmission, and blood clotting. The Dietary Reference Intake (DRI) for calcium varies with age.

Vitamin D is a fat-soluble vitamin that's naturally present in few foods. In fact, the majority of your vitamin D comes from sun exposure, which is why it's often called the sunshine vitamin. Vitamin D is essential for promoting calcium absorption in the body to keep bones and teeth strong. Ongoing research suggests vitamin D plays an important role in heart disease and cancer risk reduction as well as many other health conditions. Vitamin D deficiency is identified as an international problem. Use of sunscreen for the prevention of skin cancer has undoubtedly contributed to this issue.

Gut Facts

Because of its potential help in reducing disease, the Food and Nutrition Board experts are currently updating and reevaluating appropriate DRIs for vitamin D. The report is due in May 2010.

Calcium needs fluctuate based on age. Getting adequate calcium is key to good health, so be sure you are meeting your daily needs, as outlined in the following table.

How Much Calcium Do You Need?

Life Cycle	DRI (mg/day)
Infants:	
Birth to 6 months	210
7 months to 1 year	270
Children:	
1 to 3 years	500
4 to 8 years	800
Women:	
9 to 18 years	1,300
19 to 50 years	1,000
51 to 70+ years	1,200
Pregnant/Lactating:	
<18 years	1,300
19+ years	1,000
Men:	
9 to 18 years	1,300
19 to 50 years	1,000
51+ years	1,200

Source: National Academy of Sciences

If you are lactose intolerant, you can increase your calcium intake with these non-dairy sources of calcium:

◆ Broccoli

◆ Canned salmon with bones

◆ Fortified orange juice

◆ Green leafy vegetables

Rice and soy products, including milks, cheeses, and yogurts, often have calcium and vitamin D added with your best health in mind.

Vitamin D needs are based on adequate intake (AI) established by the Food and Nutrition Board as the amount of vitamin D sufficient to maintain bone health and normal calcium metabolism in healthy people. The following table outlines how much vitamin D (measured in International Units, or IU) you need at each stage of life.

How Much Vitamin D Do You Need?

Age	Men	Women	Pregnant/Lactating
Birth to 13 years	200 IU	200 IU	
14 to 18 years	200 IU	200 IU	200 IU
19 to 50 years	200 IU	200 IU	200 IU
51 to 70 years	400 IU	400 IU	
71+ years	600 IU	600 IU	

Source: Food and Nutrition Board

Few foods are naturally rich in vitamin D. Fattier fish such as tuna, mackerel, and salmon are good sources. Fish liver oil is a good source, but unfortunately, it contains very high amounts of vitamin A, which can be toxic to the human body. Lesser sources include egg yolks, cheese, and beef liver.

Tasty Lactose-Free Substitutes

I admit that some nondairy cheeses I've tried in the past felt rubbery and tasted quite awful. My recent adventures with cheese alternatives, however, left me pleasantly surprised.

Digestibles

Lactase enzyme supplements are available over the counter and can be taken with the first bite of dairy foods to help your body digest the lactose. Try these when you can't resist your favorite lasagna or ice cream!

Rice and soy cheese products are great substitutes for the dairy versions. Cottage cheese is available in a reduced-lactose variety. You can find reduced-lactose milk, as well, although it tastes a bit sweeter than traditional cow's milk. (The sweet flavor is due to the degradation of lactose into its digestible sugars, galactose, and glucose.) Soy milk and rice milk are also available, in plain and vanilla. Most are dairy free, but to be safe, check the ingredient list for any hidden sources of lactose.

Dairy products are a source of sugar, varying amounts of fat, and lactose—all of which can stimulate the gastrointestinal tract. So even if lactose intolerance isn't an issue, these products may pose a problem if you consume them in large quantities.

Fructose Malabsorption

Fructose, the sugar found primarily in fruits and honey, can be problematic for the IBS sufferer because *fructose malabsorption* mimics lactose intolerance.

Fructose absorption, however, doesn't require a digestive enzyme for digestion. Instead, it relies on the presence of another simple sugar, glucose, to aid its transport from the intestine into the bloodstream.

Wellness Words

Fructose is a simple sugar, known commonly as fruit sugar. **Fructose malabsorption** occurs when fructose is not properly digested in the small intestine.

Fructose Facts

All humans have limited absorption of fructose, but those with more sensitive intestines are less likely to tolerate the gas and bloating that result from excess fructose. Did you know your intestines are highly sensitive? It is estimated that only half of the population is able to completely absorb an amount of 25 grams of fructose in the diet. The average daily intake around the world ranges from 11 to 54 grams!

Even with available glucose to help absorb the fructose, the body has a point where fructose absorption is limited. Diets rich in fruits, sodas with high-fructose corn syrup (HFCS), and processed foods all contribute to an abundance of fructose in your diet. In the United States, an outrageous surge of HFCS use has increased the fructose consumption and likely has contributed to the increasing incidence of IBS. Additionally, agave syrup, which has gained recent popularity as a sweetener, has excess fructose, too.

For the IBS sufferer, with heightened sensitivity to changes in the intestine, even small amounts of fructose malabsorption may be intolerable. Some experts believe that 50 percent of those with IBS experience fructose malabsorption. Could you be one of them? Be sure to track your fructose intake by reading food labels looking for HFCS, fructose, and crystalline fructose. Also note your tolerance to fruits with excess fructose.

Beware Sources of Excess Fructose

All fruits contain fructose, and large portions can make you gassy or may make you fly for the nearest toilet. For best absorption, limit yourself to one fruit per meal or snack time. Certain fruits and foods contain more fructose than glucose and can be particularly problematic. The unabsorbed fructose becomes a food for the bacteria living in the large intestine. Gas, bloating, and diarrhea can be the not-so-lovely result.

Limit the following if fructose is a problem for you:

- Apples
- Coconut milk and coconut cream
- Dried fruit and fruit juices
- Guava
- Honey
- Mangoes

- Molasses
- Pears
- Products made with HFCS
- Sherry and port
- Watermelon

Belly-Friendly Fructose Choices

Choosing fruits that contain more glucose than fructose is your best bet for IBS management. Remember, aim to keep fruit to one portion per meal or snack.

Here are some well-tolerated fruits:

- Bananas (ripe)
- Blackberries
- Blueberries
- Cranberries
- Grapefruit
- Grapes
- Kiwifruit

- Lemons
- Limes
- Oranges
- Raspberries
- Rhubarb
- Strawberries

These fruits do not have excess fructose compared to glucose, making them more readily absorbed by the body.

What's a FODMAP?

You may think *FODMAP* is a new GPS tracking device, but it's not. FODMAP is an acronym for Fermentable Oligosaccharides, Disaccharides, *Monosaccharides*, and Polyols. Oligosaccharides are complex carbohydrates made up of multiple sugar molecules, while disaccharides are made up of two sugar molecules. FODMAPs are a collective group of carbohydrates commonly malabsorbed in the intestine, causing excess gas, bloating, and diarrhea.

We've already looked at two of the most troublesome FODMAPs, lactose and fructose. Other FODMAP groups include fructans (found in wheat), polyols (sugar alcohols), and galactans (dried peas, beans, and soy).

Wellness Words

FODMAPs are a group of fermentable carbohydrates that may contribute to gas, bloating, and diarrhea in susceptible individuals. **Monosaccharide** is a one-molecule sugar or simple sugar. Glucose (blood sugar), fructose (fruit sugar), and galactose (one of the sugars found in the milk sugar, lactose) are all monosaccharides.

Frustrating Fructans

Fructans are another group of poorly absorbed carbohydrates. They're composed of chains of the sugar fructose. Humans lack the enzyme necessary to break the fructose chains, so the fructans remain undigested in the body. They also contribute to osmotic diarrhea, as the body responds to their presence by releasing water into the intestine as they sit undigested in the large bowel.

Inulin and FOS, also known as fructooligosaccharides, are sources of fructans. Of note, there has been a recent surge of use of inulin and FOS added in various food products as a means to increase the food's fiber content. Fructan-rich foods include the following:

♦ Artichokes

♦ Asparagus

♦ Beer

♦ Garlic

♦ Leeks

♦ Onions

♦ Wheat

Wellness Words

Inulin is a dietary fiber found in a variety of foods, including wheat and onions. For people with IBS, inulin can cause gas and bloating because it's a fructan, one of the fermentable carbohydrates.

Because the American diet is so rich in wheat products, wheat is the biggest supplier of fructans in the diet. Minimizing wheat and other fructan-rich foods may be a key strategy for controlling your IBS symptoms. I find bagels particularly bothersome, but smaller bread portions such as English muffins are completely tolerable. Try choosing smaller portions of wheat-based foods and other fructan-rich foods such as onions and garlic, and assess your symptoms. If you discover wheat is a trigger for you, substitute some of your favorite wheat foods with rice, rice pasta, or alternative grains such as quinoa, millet, buckwheat (kasha), and oats.

Garlic powder and onion powder can be substituted in your favorite recipes, or use sliced onions or large chunk garlic when sautéing and then remove them prior to eating to add flavor without the added fructans.

Problems with Polyols

Polyols are known as sugar alcohols because they bear a resemblance to both sugar and alcohol in chemical structure. The problem with polyols is they cause osmotic diarrhea. Fruits naturally containing polyols include these:

- Apples
- Apricots
- Cherries
- Nectarines
- Peaches
- Pears
- Plums
- Prunes

Polyols provide a laxative effect and can be useful in the treatment of constipation. That's why prune juice is often used as a constipation remedy!

Polyols are used frequently in sugar-free products such as mints, gum, candy, and some specialty low-carbohydrate or low-sugar products. Check ingredient lists for these polyols, which may cause diarrhea:

- Isomalt
- Hydrogenated lactitol
- Lactitol
- Maltitol
- Mannitol
- Sorbitol
- Xylitol

Limiting polyols can be an important step in managing your IBS, particularly if you tend to overdo polyol-rich sugar-free candies or if you choose fruits that contain both excess fructose and polyols, such as apples, pears, and peaches.

Tummy Trouble _____

Sorbitol and maltitol are often added to sugar-free gum. You might be able to tolerate a piece or two, but if you're popping in several at a time, you may find you'll be looking for the nearest restroom soon after!

Get Away from the Galactans

Galactans are one of the oligosaccharides in the FODMAP family. Galactans contain chains of the simple sugar galactose. Galactans, just like fructans, are easily malabsorbed by the body because we lack the digestive enzyme to absorb them. In plain English, that means they're complex sugars that aren't efficiently digested.

You may want to minimize these galactan sources in your diet:

♦ Brussels sprouts

♦ Cabbage

♦ Chickpeas and hummus

♦ Kidney beans

♦ Lentils

♦ Soy products such as soy milk

♦ Veggie burgers (made with beans or soy)

♦ Wax beans

When food is malabsorbed, the same story unfolds, undigested food causes uncomfortable side effects, and—you guessed it—gas, bloating, and diarrhea. Go easy on the beans.

The Cumulative Effect

Each individual has his or her own personal threshold for FODMAP carbohydrates. Some fermentable carbohydrates may be more problematic than others for you. Some foods contain multiple FODMAP groups such as pears and apples, which contain both excess fructose and polyols.

The most important concept to understand is this: *the more FODMAPs you consume together, the more likely they will have a cumulative effect on your intestine.* You may tolerate milk in your coffee, but you might not tolerate milk and cheese at the same meal. I find that if I consume a wheat tortilla (fructans) with cheese (lactose) and beans (galactans), I really pay the price. On the other hand, eating whole-grain bread (fructans) with milk (lactose) doesn't pose any problem for me.

Assessing your tolerance and threshold for these fermentable carbohydrates is the first step to eating well with IBS. (To detail foods and symptoms, I suggest keeping a food diary—see Chapter 4.)

Gut Facts

Both lactose intolerance and fructose malabsorption can be diagnosed with hydrogen or methane breath tests. This test can be preformed at a lab, as undigested carbohydrates can lead to the formation of gases from the bacteria in the large intestine. The gas is absorbed from the intestine into the blood, where it is carried to the lungs and exhaled and measured. Measurements are made to see if the amount of gas exhaled has increased after consuming fructose or lactose.

Fiber: Friend or Foe?

Fiber is a complex carbohydrate found in plant foods that your body cannot digest. Fiber is controversial when it comes to IBS. Although in years past, it was the first-line treatment many physicians suggested, fiber has varying effects on IBS symptoms, and this general guideline of "increasing fiber" may not be appropriate in all cases.

Fiber can get your intestinal motor running too quickly. For the person with diarrhea-predominant IBS, getting the intestines moving any more is rarely the goal. For constipation-predominant IBS, however, adding fiber can be helpful.

Soluble Versus Insoluble Fiber

Fiber comes in two forms, *insoluble fiber* (not your friend), found primarily in wheat and bran, and *soluble fiber* (your best friend), found in oats and fruit. Most foods have a combination of the two types of fiber.

IBS-Friendly Fiber Sources

Although whole-wheat bread and wheat... to the diet to increase fiber content, wh...

> ✎ **Digestibles** _____
>
> Always increase fiber slowly over a few weeks to allow your body to get used to the change in your diet, and drink plenty of water to aid its movement through your intestines.

The following table offers some m...

Friendly Fiber-Rich Foods

Food	Portion
Oat bran, dry	⅓ cup
Barley, cooked	½ cup
Strawberries	1 cup
Parsnips	½ cup
Oatmeal, dry	⅓ cup
Orange	1 medium
Potato	1 medium
Winter squash	½ cup
Oatmeal bread	1 slice
Brown rice, cooked	½ cup

Source: USDA

tes cause their most trouble when combined ...DMAPs in your diet. Try your best to ...er the course of the day. Bear in mind, too, ...BS is to allow for as much variety of foods ...best-t...ore intimate with the FODMAP family, and Additi... a sour... and ce...

W... adding...ctose, fructose, fructans, galactans, and (ideall... bluebe...essential for health and intake may be as kasl...foods. produc... on your body, so limit to one fruit serving ...and control your intake as necessary for

...S compared with insoluble fiber and is ...nd beans.

Chapter 3

As a Matter of Fat

In This Chapter

- Fat and the IBS connection
- Your body's response to excess fat
- Living low fat and symptom free
- Tasty low-fat substitutes

Fats get a lot of press when it comes to heart disease and health, and we all know a diet heavy in animal fats and fatty foods is the recipe for clogged arteries. Your IBS is one more reason to stop chewin' on the fat. When it comes to IBS, too much fat in the diet can kick your body into high gear, and you don't want that.

There's no need to get overzealous here and eliminate *all* fat from your diet, because some daily fat does your body good. And let's face it—fat makes food taste good! Understanding some "fat basics" will keep your IBS in good control without sacrificing all the flavor. In this chapter, you learn where you get fat, how much fat you need for good health, and how to minimize fat in your favorite foods without losing flavor. Soon you'll be on your way to healthful, low-fat living. Your intestines will thank you.

The Role of Fats in IBS

So what's the connection between fat and IBS? Allow me one small but important science lesson: every time you eat, you stimulate your *gastrocolic reflex*. This involuntary reflex is the way your body automatically controls movements or contractions in your intestine. The gastrocolic reflex is exaggerated in IBS and often overreacts to eating. Dietary fats in particular get the gastrocolic reflex going, setting off a cascade of movements in your intestine. These movements can make you feel intestinal cramps and pain or make you urgently seek the nearest toilet. Consequently, managing your fat intake is pretty important if you want to diminish those not-so-pleasant symptoms.

Wellness Words

Gastrocolic reflex triggers intestinal movement or motility with the onset of eating.

You might find that just when you sit down to eat, your stomach gets fired up, grumbling and moving, almost like it's talking to you. That's your gastrocolic reflex in action. So while you may think the food you just ate didn't agree with you, it's more likely your overactive reflex speaking to you.

Foods rich in fats also require more stomach acid and time to be broken down for digestion. This is one of the reasons you may feel uncomfortably full following a high-fat meal.

Fats and Your Health

Although too much fat in the diet certainly gets a bad rap linked with heart disease, obesity, and even cancer risk, some daily fat does the body good. Let's take a peek at what fat can do for you:

♦ Keeps skin and hair healthy

♦ Provides fat-soluble vitamins A, D, E, and K

♦ Supplies essential fats the body is unable to make on its own

♦ Allows for proper brain development in infancy

♦ Helps insulate your organs and provides a layer of padding to keep your body warm in the wintertime

When it comes to good health and fats, most experts agree that minimizing animal fats is a good start. Although all fats have 9 calories per gram and provide the body with energy, that's where their similarity ends. Fats are often thought of as good fats and bad fats, depicting how they impact our health. Let's take a closer look at these so-called bad and good guys.

The Bad Fats

Saturated fats are considered one of the bad fats because they increase blood cholesterol, subsequently increasing your risk of heart attack or stroke. These fats are most often found in foods that are solid at room temperature or fatty animal food sources. Examples of foods rich in saturated fat are:

- Beef
- Butter
- Cheese
- Cream
- Ice cream
- Lard
- Poultry skin
- Sausage
- Whole milk

Keep these fats to a minimum in your daily diet, and your heart will be grateful. In fact, the American Heart Association suggests your saturated fat intake be no more than 7 percent of your total calorie intake. The table titled "Your Daily Fat Limit" later in this chapter offers more specifics on fat intake.

Trans fats are the unhealthiest of all the fats because they increase the artery-clogging low-density lipoprotein (LDL) cholesterol, the so-called bad cholesterol, and decrease the healthy cholesterol, known as high-density lipoprotein (HDL). For this reason, trans fats can set you up for a heart attack or stroke. Trans fats increase the risk of heart disease more than any other diet component, so avoid them as much as you can.

Wellness Words

Saturated fats are fats linked with heart disease found primarily in animal food sources. **Trans fats** are the worst dietary fat of all. They increase the risk for heart disease more than anything else in the diet.

Fortunately, trans fats are slowly shrinking out of American food products due to the labeling law instituted for trans fats in foods in 2006. For years, this dangerous fat flooded our food supply, and we ate it unknowingly. Examples of foods rich in trans fats include most commercial bakery products and fried foods. Be on the lookout for partially hydrogenated oil on ingredient lists. Where there's partially hydrogenated oil, there's trans fats!

The Good Fats

Polyunsaturated fats provide the body with essential fats it cannot make on its own, which is important for health. They help lower blood cholesterol—a good thing—but also tend to lower the good cholesterol (HDL), which is not so good. Having elevated HDL cholesterol lowers the risk of heart disease. Food manufacturers often utilize polyunsaturated fats in their products, so you likely get enough of these in a varied diet. Examples of polyunsaturated fats include corn, safflower, and sunflower oils.

> **Wellness Words**
>
> **Polyunsaturated fats** are generally liquid at room temperature and help lower blood cholesterol levels. **Omega-3 fats** are a type of the polyunsaturated fat family and provide heart-healthy benefits. **Monounsaturated fats** help reduce cholesterol levels and provide vitamin E, a powerful antioxidant and nutrient most of us could use more of for good health.

Omega-3 fats are found primarily in fatty fish such as salmon, mackerel, blue fish, and tuna. These fats tend to thin the blood and are associated with decreasing heart disease risk. For you vegetarians and others not fond of fish, you're in luck. Walnuts, flax-seeds, and arugula are good plant sources of omega-3 fats.

Monounsaturated fats are known as good fats because they help lower blood cholesterol levels yet help maintain the healthy HDL cholesterol. Examples of monounsaturated fats include olive and canola oils. Nuts and avocados are also great sources of these heart-healthy fats and provide a dose of vitamin E. Vitamin E acts as an anti-inflammatory agent and keeps the immune system healthy.

Determining Your Fat Limit

Every summer, I enjoy a fried scallop roll. I know, fried foods aren't the best health food, but hey, I live in New England, and it's a tradition! If I eat half the roll, I'm good to go, but eating the whole roll puts me over the edge—not good. Sometimes, going over the edge with both eyes open is okay, as long as you know you'll likely pay a bit for your dietary indiscretion. I know it's not always easy to follow all the rules, *all* the time.

There's no set fat limit for IBS, as everyone's body is different, but using the American Heart Association (AHA) guide to limiting fat in healthy people is a good starting point to appreciating your daily fat goal. According to the AHA, no more than 30 percent of your day's total calories should come from total fat. Of that, 7 percent or less should be from saturated fat and less than 1 percent should be trans fat.

The following table breaks it all down. Calorie needs are based on a number of factors, including height, weight, gender, age, and exercise level. Most women fall in the 1,200- to 1,800-calorie range, while most men, 2,000 calories and above.

Your Daily Fat Limit

Daily Calorie Needs	Total Fat	Saturated Fat	Trans Fat
1,200	<40 grams	<9 grams	<1.3 grams
1,500	<50 grams	<12 grams	<1.7 grams
1,800	<60 grams	<14 grams	<2.0 grams
2,000	<67 grams	<16 grams	<2.2 grams
2,200	<73 grams	<17 grams	<2.4 grams
2,500	<83 grams	<19 grams	<2.7 grams

With IBS, fat is best tolerated in small increments throughout the day, versus saving up your fat grams for one big power meal.

Reading nutrition facts labels will reveal the fat content in many foods. Be sure to note how much of the food you're eating compared to the serving size listed on the label. For instance, you may eat 2 cups of macaroni and cheese when the serving size is only 1 cup. In this instance, you'd have to calculate your fat intake as twice the amount listed on the food label because you ate two times the serving size.

Fats in foods vary. Try not to get too bogged down with all the number-crunching but put your effort into becoming more aware of how much fat is found in your favorite foods (the following table will help!), and modify your intake based on your symptoms related to their consumption.

Do yourself a favor and become a fat-finding detective. Read the nutrition facts labels, focusing on the total fat listed.

(U.S. Food and Drug Administration CFSAN/Office of Nutritional Products, Labeling and Dietary Supplements)

Nutrition Facts

Serving Size 1 cup (228g)
Servings Per Container 2

Amount Per Serving

Calories 250   Calories from Fat 110

	% Daily Value*
Total Fat 12g	18%
Saturated Fat 3g	15%
Trans Fat 1.5g	
Cholesterol 30mg	10%
Sodium 470mg	20%
Total Carbohydrate 31g	10%
Dietary Fiber 0g	0%
Sugars 5g	
Protein 5g	

Vitamin A	4%
Vitamin C	2%
Calcium	20%
Iron	4%

* Percent Daily Values are based on a 2,000 calorie diet. Your Daily Values may be higher or lower depending on your calorie needs:

	Calories:	2,000	2,500
Total Fat	Less than	65g	80g
Sat Fat	Less than	20g	25g
Cholesterol	Less than	300mg	300mg
Sodium	Less than	2,400mg	2,400mg
Total Carbohydrate		300g	375g
Dietary Fiber		25g	30g

Fat Found in Common Foods

Food	Portion Size	Fat
Beverages:		
Whole milk	1 cup	8 grams
Cappuccino	1½ cups	3.5 grams
Skim milk	1 cup	.4 gram
Black Coffee/tea	1 cup	0 gram
Breads:		
Blueberry muffin	1 large	26 grams
Croissant	1 medium	12 grams
Waffle	1 frozen	3.2 grams
Bagel	1 medium	1.4 grams

Food	Portion Size	Fat
Whole-wheat	1 slice	.9 gram
Cereals:		
Granola	½ cup	6.2 grams
Puffed rice	1 cup	.2 gram
Corn flakes	1 cup	.1 gram
Cheeses:		
Cheddar	1 ounce	9.4 grams
American	1 ounce	8.9 grams
Mozzarella	1 ounce	4.5 grams
Parmesan, grated	1 tablespoon	1.4 grams
Meats:		
Hamburger, regular	3 ounces	17.6 grams
Porterhouse steak	3 ounces	16.3 grams
Pork chop, center cut	3 ounces	6.2 grams
Chicken skinless breast	3 ounces	3 grams
Fish:		
Salmon	3 ounces	7 grams
Swordfish	3 ounces	4.4 grams
Tuna, canned in water	3 ounces	2.5 grams
Fats:		
Salad dressing	2 tablespoons	17 grams
Olive oil	1 tablespoon	13.5 grams
Mayo	1 tablespoon	11.7 grams
Butter	1 tablespoon	11.5 grams
Margarine	1 tablespoon	11.5 grams
Mayo, reduced-fat	1 tablespoon	4.8 grams

continues

Fat Found in Common Foods (continued)

Food	Portion Size	Fat
Desserts:		
Ice cream, rich	½ cup	17 grams
Angel food cake	1 slice	.2 gram

Source: USDA, www.nal.usda.gov, and starbucks.com

Managing Your Fat Threshold

We all have our own tolerance of fat. You'll find that a certain amount of fat works for your body, and a bit more than that really doesn't work. Keeping a food diary (see Chapter 4) can assist you in detecting your symptoms associated with the different foods you eat. As you become more aware of the fat in your diet and its impact on how you feel, you can better appreciate your personal fat threshold.

Tummy Trouble

Fast foods got you down? It's no wonder, when large french fries and a deluxe burger together contain 70 grams of fat! That's more than most people's daily quota, all in one meal.

America's favorite fatty foods are available for the taking in almost every town, on every corner. Americans really know how to fill up on fat with the classics such as burgers and fries, Philly cheese steaks, fisherman's platters, and meatloaf with mashed potatoes and gravy. And let's not forget apple pie, which alone would be enough, but we ramp up the fat by adding a scoop of ice cream. Would you like that à la mode? Why yes, of course. Yikes!

Consuming smaller fatty food portions, and of course, with less regularity, is a good way to begin lowering your fat intake. Begin substituting lower-fat alternatives for your full-fat favorites. This is rather easy to do because lower-fat foods have come a long way in taste and availability.

More on dining out and IBS to come in Chapter 8, but to get you started, here are some simple tips to curb the fat when dining out:

◆ Order milk in your coffee and say no to cream.

◆ Opt for mustard on your sandwiches and hold the mayo!

◆ Pass on the beef, and order chicken or fish instead.

- ◆ Try the turkey sandwich instead of the pastrami.

- ◆ Hold the french fries and opt for the baked potato.

- ◆ Say yes to grilled or baked meat and say no way to fried.

- ◆ Order the kiddy cone and resist the sundae!

Balancing your low-fat menu choices with a high-fat treat can be a good strategy when you crave a fat-filled, indulgent food. Opt to eat a low-fat meal of grilled chicken, green beans, a baked potato, and then—ta-da!—treat yourself to a small piece of fudge chocolate cake.

Alternatively, you could overdo it, with the large steak, french fries, broccoli with cheese sauce, and no-you-shouldn't-have-it chocolate cake. At the end of *this* day, you might not want to have your cake and eat it, too! Of course, if you do indulge in the cake following a fatty meal such as this, you will likely kick your gastrocolic reflux into overdrive. I bet you won't do that two days in a row.

Great Low-Fat Recipe Replacements

Reducing fat in your beloved family recipes can be quite simple. Try to replace one or two high-fat ingredients with their lower-fat counterparts. First, try cutting fat by choosing lower-fat dairy foods. You don't have to go overboard and make more than one or two substitutions because your end product may be a well-intended flop!

The following table shows you some almost-effortless tips to help you slice some of the fat right off the top.

Recipe Makeovers

If a Recipe Calls for This ...	Substitute This ...
1 cup whole milk	1 cup buttermilk or low-fat milk
1 cup heavy cream	1 cup evaporated milk
1 cup cheese	1 cup reduced-fat cheese
2 tablespoons oil for sauté	2 tablespoons broth or wine
$\frac{1}{2}$ cup brown gravy	$\frac{1}{2}$ cup beef broth thickened with cornstarch
2 whole eggs	4 egg whites or $\frac{1}{2}$ cup egg substitute

continues

Recipe Makeovers (continued)

If a Recipe Calls for This ...	Substitute This ...
1 cup chocolate chips	½ cup chocolate chips and ½ cup oatmeal
1 pound ground beef	1 pound ground turkey or chicken breast
5 slices bacon	5 slices turkey bacon or Canadian bacon

Reducing Fat in Your Food

By now you understand that too much fat in your IBS diet may trigger unwanted symptoms. And that's not all. We know too much fat in the diet is linked with health problems such as cancer, heart disease, and gastric reflux. Trimming the fat from your diet may offer more health benefits than you can imagine.

Gut Facts

Heart disease remains America's number-one cause of death. High blood cholesterol levels increase your risk. Remember, there's good cholesterol and bad cholesterol? Good cholesterol is HDL—let the *H* remind you that it's *healthful.* LDL, conversely, is the bad cholesterol; let the *L* remind you that it's *lousy.*

Swapping high-fat food options for lower-fat alternatives is easy when you find yummy substitutes. There is some evidence that your body will adapt to the lower-fat foods and they'll become your preferred choices. I know firsthand: when I first tried milk in coffee, I wasn't sure I'd like the change. Now, I can't stand tasting even a bit of cream in my coffee. See how your body adapts to healthier, lower-fat fare. Start making your low-fat swaps using the following table as a guide.

Great Food Swaps to Lower-Fat Content

Instead of This High-Fat Food ...	Substitute This ...
Bacon, pork	Canadian bacon
Beef	Chicken or fish
Bologna/salami	Turkey or ham
Cheese	Reduced-fat cheese
Chocolate ice cream	Fudgesicle

Instead of This High-Fat Food ...	Substitute This ...
Creamed sauce	Wine or broth sauce
Hamburger	Grilled chicken
Potato chips	Baked chips
Potato chips	Pretzels
Pound cake	Angel food cake
Whole milk	1 percent or skim milk

Limiting fat in your diet will likely help manage your IBS symptoms while lowering your risk of other chronic diseases. Remember, all healthy diets should regularly include a bit of good, healthful fats such as olive oil, nuts, seeds, and fish.

The Least You Need to Know

◆ Too much fat aggravates your IBS by stimulating the gastrocolic reflux.

◆ Choose grilling, baking over frying to minimize fats in your diet without compromising flavor.

◆ Fat comes in heart-healthy varieties such as olive oil and canola oil, fatty fish, and nuts and seeds. Less-heart-healthy fats can be found in commercially baked goods and fried foods.

◆ Everybody needs fat for good health because it helps our body absorb fat-soluble vitamins A, D, E, and K. Fat is essential for keeping our skin and hair healthy, too.

◆ Substitute high-fat foods with low-fat alternatives as an easy first step to lowering fat.

Chapter 4

Could You Have a Food Intolerance or Allergy?

In This Chapter

- ◆ Understanding food intolerance, sensitivity, and allergy
- ◆ Comparing gluten sensitivity and toxic gluten reaction
- ◆ A look at histamine intolerance
- ◆ The role of a food diary

Food allergies are at an all-time high these days. I bet you know at least one child with a peanut allergy, or maybe two or three. Food intolerance, food sensitivity, and food allergies are often thought to mean the same thing, but each involves very different processes in the body. Understanding the potential connection between your IBS and food reactions is another important step in eating well with IBS.

In this chapter, you learn to recognize the differences among food intolerance, allergies, and sensitivities. IBS sufferers are likely to have food-related issues, so appreciating how food can impact your body is essential. Keeping a food diary and charting your symptoms is also useful in uncovering problematic foods.

Food Allergy Versus Intolerance

A *food allergy* is an immune system response to food, usually to the protein component, and the body mistakes the food as harmful. Reactions to food involving the immune system can be immediate or have a delayed response. Some can be life-threatening. Severe allergic reactions to food are called anaphylaxis. These reactions can lead to breathing difficulties and shock with the potential of death.

Food allergy is a rapidly growing public health problem. In fact, from 1997 to 2002, the number of peanut allergies *doubled*. No wonder you know someone with a peanut allergy! An estimated 4 to 8 percent of children and 2 percent of adults in the United States have food allergies.

Gut Facts

The Food Allergy and Anaphylaxis Network is a great resource for food allergies. Check out www.foodallergy.org for recipes, traveling tips, allergy facts, and much more.

According to the Food Allergy and Anaphylaxis Network, 8 foods account for 90 percent of all food allergies:

- Eggs
- Fish
- Milk
- Peanuts

- Shellfish
- Soy
- Tree nuts
- Wheat

In 2004, the Food and Drug Administration instituted the Food Labeling and Consumer Protection Act requiring that foods that contain any of the top eight *allergens* have them labeled in bold on the ingredient list. The law was instituted for all foods labeled on or after January 1, 2006. You may recall having seen bold letters following the ingredients list on food items revealing the allergens in the product.

With food allergy reactions, a chain of events occur in the body after exposure to a food the body deems toxic. The reaction of the immune system to food allergens follows this sequence of events:

1. The immune system recognizes the food as an allergen, or invader.

2. The body classifies the allergen as dangerous.

3. The body responds by making *antibodies* to stop the invasion of this perceived dangerous allergen.

Approximately 60 percent of IBS sufferers believe food contributes to their symptoms, and research has shown that food allergy could trigger IBS symptoms. Adults with seasonal allergies, eczema, and asthma are more likely to report IBS symptoms, suggesting a possible link of allergy with IBS symptoms in some individuals.

Scientific evidence in the study of food allergy and IBS is just emerging, and no definitive goals or recommendations have been established for allergy testing for those with IBS. Because treatment for IBS is very individual, explore allergy testing if you and your physician feel it's warranted.

Unlike life-threatening allergic reactions, *food intolerance* and *sensitivities* do not pose serious risk. Often food intolerance occurs when the body lacks an enzyme to properly digest a particular food. Food intolerance and food sensitivities are common in IBS and do warrant a further look. Lactose intolerance, for example, is prevalent in IBS and leads to digestive complaints such as diarrhea, abdominal pain, and bloating.

The science of food and the immune system is complicated stuff! Understanding the different terminology helps you differentiate among allergy, intolerance, and sensitivity. With that in mind, here are some terms you should know:

- A *food sensitivity* occurs when your body responds adversely to food. Some food sensitivities cause migraine headaches, or eczema, a dry, itchy skin rash.

- *Food allergy* is the reaction of your body's immune system to a food, usually protein-containing foods, and your body recognizes the food as foreign.

- *Food intolerance* is a negative reaction to food that does not involve the immune system, but often involves the digestive system. Lactose intolerance is one example.

- *Anaphylaxis* is a life-threatening reaction that occurs in a true food allergy and can lead to breathing problems or shock.

- An *allergen* is a molecule your body recognizes as foreign or dangerous.

- *Antibodies* are molecules produced by the body in response to what it perceives as intruders or foreign substances.

Food intolerances and allergies can contribute to gastrointestinal complaints. Be sure to discuss any concerns you may have regarding potential food intolerances or allergies with your physician.

Gluten Sensitivity Versus Celiac Disease

Gluten is the protein found in wheat, rye, and barley. The gluten-free diet has gained popularity lately, touted as a cure-all for many conditions, even weight management. Unfortunately, a gluten-free diet can cause weight gain in some, and it can be a costly diet that requires educational intervention from a registered dietitian to ensure it's followed carefully to meet nutritional requirements.

Experts have found, however, that some people, including those with IBS, may have some degree of *gluten intolerance or sensitivity*. This is believed to occur when consuming gluten-containing food causes gastrointestinal distress. A number of individuals with IBS experience relief when following a gluten-free diet. When you fill out your food diary (more on that coming up later in this chapter), take note of any symptoms associated with gluten intake. Remember, any food that contains wheat, rye, and barley contains gluten. You may find minimizing or eliminating gluten can be helpful.

 Tummy Trouble

Wheat contains both fructans and gluten and is one of the common triggers for those with IBS. You may tolerate some wheat, so start reducing your wheat portions first and assess your symptoms.

Here are some common sources of gluten:

- Bread
- Breaded chicken and meats
- Breakfast cereal such as wheat- and bran-based choices
- Chocolate malt–flavored beverages (contains barley)
- Communion host/bread
- Cookies
- Crackers
- Pasta
- Pizza
- Pretzels
- Soy sauce

Celiac disease (CD), in contrast, is an *autoimmune disease* in which gluten is *toxic* to the small intestine, causing damage to the intestine. The treatment for CD is a gluten-free diet for life. Symptoms of gluten intolerance and celiac disease can be identical and include diarrhea, gas, bloating, vomiting, constipation, nausea, skin irritation, weight loss, and fatigue. Gluten intolerance or sensitivity, conversely, does not cause any known damage to the intestines.

Wellness Words

Gluten is the general name for the storage proteins found in wheat, rye, and barley. **Gluten intolerance or sensitivity** occurs when your body reacts negatively to gluten in the diet. An **autoimmune disease** is one that occurs when your immune system is overreactive and your body actually attacks itself. **Celiac disease** (CD) is an autoimmune disease in which gluten ingestion is toxic to the intestines

IBS is a fairly common condition, affecting about 10 out of 100 people in the United States. At present, celiac disease occurs in about 1 out of 100 people in the United States—a rate similar to many European countries. Recent studies reviewing incidence of celiac disease in people with IBS suggest that those with IBS were four times more likely to have celiac disease compared to healthy individuals.

The American College of Gastroenterology Task Force recommends that people with diarrhea-predominant IBS, or IBS that fluctuates between diarrhea and constipation, be screened for celiac disease. Initial screening for CD can be done with a blood test at your doctor's office. In order for the test to be accurate, you must be eating a gluten-rich diet regularly when tested. The gold standard test for celiac disease requires multiple biopsies of the small intestine.

For more on the gluten-free diet and celiac disease, see Appendix B or check out the Celiac Disease Foundation's website at www.celiac.org.

Heard About Histamine?

We know lactose intolerance is fairly common and results from the lack of the enzyme lactase. Well, here's another food intolerance I would like to introduce to you. *Histamine intolerance* is an inability to break down the histamine found in many foods due to inadequate amounts of the enzyme diamine oxidase (DAO).

Histamine is a protein found in a variety of foods, particularly weekend-splurge foods such as beer, pizza, and wine! The histamine content of food increases the longer the food is exposed to microbes such as in the processing of alcohol and cheeses, so these are big sources of histamine.

Some foods are naturally high in histamine:

- Eggplant
- Pumpkin
- Sauerkraut
- Spinach
- Tomato and tomato products

Symptoms of histamine intolerance include diarrhea, headache, asthma, and hives. If you think you may have histamine intolerance, discuss your symptoms with your doctor.

Keeping a Food Diary

A food diary can be a terrific tool to help you uncover problematic foods. The more details you note in your diary, the more valuable it will be to you and your doctor.

How and where you keep your food diary is up to you. Use whatever system you're most comfortable with and you will, indeed, use. You could keep an actual pen-and-paper diary in a notebook, create a more elaborate Excel spreadsheet on your computer, or anything in between.

What Should I Keep Track Of?

Ultimately the level of detail you keep is up to you, but for best results I recommend you include the following in your food diary:

- Everything you eat and drink, including gum, mints, the chocolate on your co-worker's desk—*everything!*
- Timing of meals and timing of symptoms.
- Ingredients you include in your recipes such as spices or added fats.
- Medications you take and their ingredients, when provided.

Digestibles _____

Commenting on your symptoms and severity in your food diary provides a better indication of what foods you tolerate and don't tolerate. Be sure to also include the time of day you ate, which may help you uncover delayed food reactions versus quick assaults, such as lactose intolerance, which usually occurs within two hours of ingestion.

When you begin your food diary, continue eating all the foods you normally eat, and note your resulting symptoms along with a rating of the severity of your symptoms. Here are some handy keys to help you keep track:

Symptoms:

- D—diarrhea/frequency
- C—constipation
- B—bloating
- P—pain
- G—gas

Severity:

- 0—no symptoms
- 1—symptoms are mild
- 2—symptoms are uncomfortable but manageable
- 3—symptoms are unbearable

If you uncover certain problematic foods, remove them from your diet for a week and reassess your symptoms. Do you feel better? If you still feel there's room for improvement, consider minimizing lactose or another FODMAP group (remember FODMAPs from Chapter 2?). The goal is to allow for variety in your diet while minimizing your symptoms.

You might also want to rate how you feel on a scale from 1 to 10. Let 10 be your best and 1 be miserable. Work your way to 10 to feel your best.

 Tummy Trouble _____

The American College of Gastroenterology does not support the use of elimination diets in IBS management at this time, but some nutrition experts find use of elimination diets very constructive. Following an elimination diet should be done with the help of a skilled dietitian, as there are many different types of elimination diets and many are limited from a nutritional perspective and therefore should be utilized for short periods of time. Working closely with your physician and dietitian can help you determine if a trial of an elimination diet is appropriate for you.

The Benefits of Keeping Track

When you become more aware of your diet and its impact on how you feel, you'll have the information you need to start incorporating change. For example, in my practice, I had a client with IBS who had continued gas despite removing dairy products from her diet. After evaluating her intake for a week, she uncovered that every time she ate hummus and apples, she felt gassy. Uncovering what foods trigger your personal symptoms is key for feeling and eating well with IBS.

Additionally, if you track your intake with the help of a registered dietitian (R.D.)—which I highly recommend you do—you can gain insight into your trigger foods as well as the overall nutritional balance of your diet. A registered dietitian is trained in detecting nutritional shortcomings.

It's very common to believe that your diet is better than it really is. It's not very helpful, though, so visualizing your intake in black and white is a great tool to truly see what you're doing right and what you could do better.

More Noteworthy Considerations

In addition to tracking your food triggers, consider the following points:

Do you have fruits and vegetables present at every meal?

Have you included calcium-rich foods—dairy products, fortified orange juice, green leafy vegetables, canned salmon with bones, broccoli, etc.—to keep your bones and teeth healthy?

Do you have a variety of different-color fruits and vegetables? Something green, red, orange, white, purple, and/or blue? The pigment in the skin of fruits and vegetables provides various health benefits—one more great reason for variety!

Any nuts in your diet? Nuts are a terrific source of protein and magnesium. Studies have shown nuts in the diet lower the risk of heart disease. Keep nut portions to the serving size listed on the food label because they're high in fat, which can trigger IBS.

Do you choose heart-healthy oils such as canola and olive oil?

Do you opt for healthy protein foods—chicken, lean beef, fish, low-fat cheeses and yogurt, nuts or nut butters, beans, and legumes (depending on tolerance)—and include them at most or all meals and snack times?

Are your grains whole or refined? Whole grains offer more fiber and nutrients. White flour is refined, while whole oats, brown rice, and whole-wheat products are whole grains.

Keying in to how food reacts in your body helps you uncover the foods that work best in your body. Now get going and start tracking your intake!

The Least You Need to Know

- ◆ People with IBS are four times more likely to be diagnosed with celiac disease than non-IBS sufferers.

- ◆ Experts recommend people with diarrhea-predominant IBS or those who alternate between diarrhea and constipation be screened for celiac disease.

- ◆ Food allergies can be life-threatening, while food intolerances and sensitivities are not.

- ◆ Food intolerance and sensitivities are common in IBS and often include lactose intolerance and gluten sensitivity.

- ◆ Keeping a food diary is a great tool to assess your tolerance to foods.

Chapter 5

Your Best Digestion Lifestyle

In This Chapter

- Your digestion and how IBS affects it
- Importance of making time to eat
- Large food portions = digestive woes
- Gum, straw use, and soda and belly bloating
- Understanding alcohol and caffeine moderation

Find yourself eating in your car lately? How about those in-between-meeting gulps? Life seems to have become busier, and while children seem to have less time to eat at school lunchtime, it seems adults often find it difficult to find time for a calm, relaxing meal as well. These rushed, stress-filled eating experiences can negatively impact the way you chew your foods (who has time to chew?). Also affected is your stress level, which ultimately affects your body's ability to adequately digest the foods you eat.

If you slam into your morning with a big cup of coffee and end it with a few cocktails, you might find this lifestyle isn't quite working for your sad intestines. In this chapter, we unravel how your body digests foods, and how you can help your body absorb foods better. You'll uncover the amount of caffeine and alcohol in your diet and better understand your personal threshold.

Digestion 101

Digestion begins in the mouth. Chewing properly is the first step to healthy digestion. While you chew, *amylase*, a digestive enzyme, is released in the mouth and initiates the breakdown of carbohydrates. This is an important step in your digestive process because some carbohydrates are poorly digested in IBS.

From your mouth and down your esophagus, food makes its way to your stomach, where additional enzymes and stomach acid break down protein and fat into smaller components. From there, the food travels to the small intestine, where the pancreas releases even more enzymes to aid digestion. Next stop is the small intestine, where more enzymes are released, breaking complex sugars into single-molecule absorbable sugars. This is where the food is absorbed into the bloodstream. The large intestine is responsible for absorbing excess water back into the body and helping form stool.

Wellness Words

Amylase is a digestive enzyme released in the mouth to help break down carbohydrates.

These are all very important steps to absorbing food properly and minimizing the risk for malabsorption, which contributes to symptoms of IBS. You see, your body is a very busy machine making food become energy so you can move about and live your life!

Proper digestion involves your entire digestive tract.

(nih.gov)

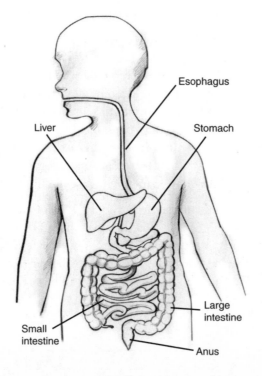

Esophagus

Liver

Stomach

Large intestine

Small intestine

Anus

Growing up as the youngest in a family of nine children, dinnertime was a time in my life where survival of the fittest took on real meaning. If you considered having a second helping, you better be the first to finish the *first* serving. Growing up this way has created a natural inclination for me to eat fast. Knowing that's not the best practice for my health, I try to slow down and take adequate time to chew my food and relax while I eat.

Do you think you may be a fast eater, too? To maximize your digestion, be sure to make time for slow, relaxing mealtimes.

Chew On This!

Slowing down and chewing properly are important aspects of digestion. By chewing food, you expose more of the food's surface area to the enzymes present in your mouth. As more of the food is exposed to the enzymes, it's broken down more effectively. The saliva in your mouth also softens the food so it can slide down your esophagus to your stomach easily.

Ever swallow a sharp tortilla chip or cracker the wrong way? Ouch! If you answered yes, you could learn a thing or two about how to chew your foods correctly! Here are a few tips to help you slow down and chew:

- Put down your fork or spoon between bites.
- Try to chew your food to a paste consistency.
- Play soft music while you eat to help slow you down.
- Sip water between bites.

Savor What You Eat

Make mealtimes something you want to take time to enjoy. While at home, try simply lighting a candle, dimming the lights, or putting on soft music, which will provide indicators to your body that it's time to relax.

When my husband drives home from work, he can see the candle lit in our kitchen from the road as he approaches the house. This is his signal that our house is calm (not always the case with three kids!), and that helps calm and prepare his body to enjoy a nice meal. It's not always possible to make every meal a peaceful journey, but do try to make time for more relaxing meals as part of your healthy digestive lifestyle.

Enjoy the foods you eat, too! Food should be savored. There's some evidence that your body actually absorbs nutrients from food best when you enjoy the food you eat. Take a moment to reflect on your favorite foods and incorporate them more into your menu planning. (More on menu planning in Chapter 7.)

Digestibles

Feeling stressed? *The Relaxation Response* (Harper Paperbacks, 2000) by medical doctor Herbert Benson provides great strategies for breathing techniques to help calm you. Check it out!

Perilous Portions

You know the scenario: you're in a lunch meeting with all the "wrong" foods, you indulge, and moments later you feel your belly initiating a full-blown assault. Dining out may lead to the same scenario.

We all know portion sizes have increased over the years—just compare the size of your grandmother's china to the dish size provided at your nearest restaurant! The National Heart, Lung, and Blood Institute offers a "portion distortion" quiz on its website (www.nhlbi.nih.gov). It reveals the calorie difference in portions today compared to 20 years ago. The following table shares a few examples.

Portions from Yesteryear to Present

Food/Serving	Calories 20 Years Ago	Calories Today
Plate of spaghetti	500	1,025
French fries	210	610
Hamburger	333	590
Muffin	210	500
Bagel	140	350
Soda	85	250

Source: hin.nhlbi.nih.gov/portion/index.htm

Overeating and IBS rarely work well together. A lot of food at one given time is often too much for your intestine to handle, resulting in diarrhea and bloating. In

America, you'll find large portion sizes (coinciding with larger waistlines) more often than not, and that can make dining out with IBS a challenge.

To help minimize tummy woes that result from eating out, try to split a meal or order an appetizer-size portion. As you already know, small, frequent meals are best tolerated in IBS. (For more tips on dining out with IBS, turn to Chapter 8.) And to balance your plate and keep portions reasonable, visualize these tips:

◆ Keep your meat portion to the size of a deck of cards.

◆ Portions of carbohydrate-rich foods such as pasta, rice, potatoes, bread, peas, and corn should resemble the size of your fist.

◆ Fill half of your plate with tolerated fruits and vegetables such as a green salad, orange slices, green beans, or zucchini.

Becoming overhungry is a recipe for disaster for the IBS sufferer. When we get overhungry, we often overeat, choose less-nutritious food choices, and eat quickly, sometimes forgetting to chew thoroughly.

Set aside time in your busy schedule to eat meals at regularly arranged intervals. Don't ever skip meals. Consider getting up 15 minutes earlier to allow for a quiet breakfast. Schedule time in your work calendar for lunch. Bringing a snack with you at all times can be helpful when your schedule changes on quick notice. I always have a granola bar or nuts handy to avoid the impulsive, on-the-run junk-food purchase. Making eating right a priority in your everyday life will pay off for you.

Digestibles _____

To keep portions appropriate at home, make what you and your family should eat—no more and no less. For instance, don't make a full pound of pasta or five baked potatoes for two people. When baking cookies, bake two cookies per person and freeze the rest of the dough. If you have extra food available, it may be difficult to keep your portions in check.

Don't Eat on the Run

As crazy as this may sound, many people eat meals in their vehicle on a regular basis. Try your best not to do this. Fast-food choices have become somewhat healthier, yet they still fall short on overall good nutrition. In addition, how can you truly relax eating a meal while in rush-hour traffic?

The habit of eating in the car coincided with the arrival of the first drive-thru fast-food restaurants. In an effort to streamline our time constraints, drive-thru restaurants seem, for some, to be the answer to meal planning. McDonald's feeds more than 47 million people per day worldwide—needless to say, fast food is big business! It's no wonder we're all, globally, getting fatter, feeling fatigued, and suffering more digestive woes!

If you must eat a quick snack in the car, try to pull over and find a quiet, safe place to relax a moment and eat. On long car rides, don't rely on fast-food restaurants to feed you and your family. Pack a car picnic, and your IBS body will be grateful. By packing your lunch versus grabbing fast food, the good nutrition payback is priceless, as the following table shows.

Typical Fast-Food Meal	Picnic Lunch
Cheeseburger	Turkey sandwich
Medium french fries	Baked potato chips
Medium soda	Water bottle
Apple pie	Grapes (18)
	Baby carrots
Total calories and fat grams:	
1,140 calories, 44 grams fat	425 calories, 3.5 grams fat

By choosing to pack your lunch instead of eating a typical fast-food meal, you saved 715 calories and 40.5 grams of fat—and likely ate more fruit and vegetables, too! You probably even saved a few bucks.

Brown-bagging in general is a good idea because you have better control over what you eat. When you dine out, it's easy to impulsively choose less-healthful food options. Plus, if you don't really enjoy what's available but eat it anyway, you'll likely be looking for other food items soon after your meal because your cravings weren't satisfied.

Adding Air: Gum, Soda, and Straws

As a former gum chewer and carbonated-beverage-drinking queen, I can tell you from experience: these habits may set you up for a gas-filled belly. Add a straw to the beverage, and the situation could go from bad to worse.

IBS sufferers have enough gas and bloating to contend with already. Adding more air via straw use or drinking carbonated beverages can be painful. It's not that you should never chew gum, but be aware that chewing gum with carbonated beverages or long-term chewing alone can make you feel bloated like a balloon! Most restaurants offer a straw even with a glass of water. Remove the straw and sip from the glass to minimize the air you're sucking directly into your belly.

 Tummy Trouble _____

Sugar-free gum often contains polyols, in the form of sugar alcohols such as sorbitol or maltitol, which can contribute to gas, bloating, and diarrhea.

Today, carbonated beverage consumption is at an all-time high. Soda in America is most often sweetened with high-fructose corn syrup (HFCS). That HFCS often has a fairly even amount of glucose in it, allowing the fructose to be absorbed adequately. So a glass of soda is often tolerated with IBS. Larger amounts, however, may be a problem for two reasons: one the carbonation, and two, the body can only handle so much fructose in a day! So don't go reaching for the 2-liter bottle.

No one has more control over what goes in your mouth than you. Habits, food favorites, lifestyle, and your schedule all affect your food and beverage choices. Unfortunately, with IBS, too much of a *good* thing can become a bad thing. If you must indulge, keep to the motto, "All things in moderation."

Alcohol: When Happy Hour Isn't So Happy

Enjoying a cocktail to commemorate the weekend or a special event is a celebratory and sensible indulgence. When the merrymaking becomes more generous, and comments such as "Yes, we'll have another round of drinks," are repeated, payback will likely ensue for the person with IBS. Too much alcohol and IBS don't make a happy pair.

Alcohol interferes with adequate absorption of water from the intestines, complicated by excess water being released into the intestine. These events combine and result in watery diarrhea for some folks. Sounds lovely, doesn't it? Too much alcohol is also linked with heartburn, as alcohol can irritate the stomach lining. That's just one more reason to keep the cocktails to a minimum if you have IBS (or even if you don't!).

For you wheat-sensitive folks, bear in mind that beer contains wheat ingredients and is known to be particularly bothersome for those with IBS. Besides, carbonated beverages can cause bloating, so consider avoiding them when ordering your cocktail of choice. The important take-away here: know your body and its limits!

Alcohol and Your Health

Alcohol manufacturers point to a slew of research claiming alcohol is good for heart health. Experts have linked moderate alcohol consumption to decreased risk of sudden death and lower risk of heart disease. And even the French, despite their heavy use of butter and cheese, seem to derive heart benefits from the red wine they enjoy. (Their decadency has been coined the "French paradox" because the French have a low rate of heart disease despite their rich diet.)

Wellness Words

Cirrhosis of the liver involves a slow deterioration of liver function and healthy liver tissue becomes scarred. Cirrhosis has a number of causes, among them infections, toxins, and alcohol abuse.

But there truly is another side of the coin when it comes to alcohol and your health. High alcohol intake can lead to dementia, colon and breast cancer, *cirrhosis* of the liver, and alcoholism.

Keeping It Moderate

The key message here is keep your alcohol intake *moderate*. For some of my clients, moderate consumption, in their opinion, is six beers on a Saturday night! Sorry to say, that doesn't fit the criteria for moderation!

What is moderate intake? About one drink per day for women and two drinks per day for men. Check out the following table to see how much of your favorite drink adds up to one serving of alcohol.

What's Considered One Drink?

Type of Alcohol	Quantity
Hard liquor (distilled spirits)	$1\frac{1}{2}$ ounces
Beer	12 ounces
Wine	5 ounces

The alcohol content of a beverage is noted by its proof, which is two times the alcohol content. For instance, Bacardi 151 proof is 75.5 percent alcohol. Alcohol by volume (ABV) may be stated on a bottle; this refers to how much of the total volume of liquid is alcohol. The higher the proof, the more alcohol, the more effect the drink will have on your IBS and state of mind!

Sensible Solutions

Some IBS sufferers find carbonated cocktails or beer products with wheat ingredients less tolerable than pure distilled spirits or a glass of wine. Frozen concoctions often have syrups and sugars made of HFCS, which as you know can be unsettling to the IBS belly. Avoid drinks with coconut milk such as piña coladas, as well as sherries and ports, all of which contain FODMAPs.

If you must partake in the celebrating, try one of these better-tolerated options and assess your tolerance:

- ◆ 5 ounces red or white wine
- ◆ 1½ ounces vodka with orange juice
- ◆ 12 ounces gluten-free beer
- ◆ 5 ounces wine spritzer

Caffeine Confusion

With a coffee shop on almost every block, I think it's fair to say we love our java! Our caffeine comes in many forms, but coffee seems to be our biggest source. Chocolate, tea, energy drinks, and some soda come with a dose of caffeine. I have to admit, I love my coffee. But too much of it makes me feel awful.

The key to mixing caffeine and IBS is learning your limit. Caffeine is a drug that acts as a stimulant in your body. As such, it can stimulate or increase the movement of the intestines. For some constipation-predominant IBS sufferers, that can be the ticket to success; for others, with more diarrhea-predominant IBS, not so much!

 Tummy Trouble

The recent surge of caffeine drinks paired with alcohol has prompted concern, as studies have shown those who combine these products are more likely to be involved in alcohol-related injuries.

Countless studies have been done on caffeine and health, and the final consensus is that moderate amounts of caffeine appear to be safe. In some cases, modest caffeine intake may lower risk of ovarian cancer and diabetes.

Hidden Sources of Caffeine

Obvious sources of caffeine are coffee, tea, and cola, but caffeine sneaks into our diet in many other products, such as chocolate, cocoa, energy drinks, and even some aspirin products. Do you know how much caffeine you're consuming? Take a closer look at some of your favorite drinks and even some medications that provide a kick of caffeine.

Caffeine Content for Drinks and More

Item	Serving Size	Caffeine
Drinks:		
Starbucks coffee, Pikes Place Roast	16 ounces (grande)	330 milligrams
Monster Energy	16 ounces	160 milligrams
Red Bull	8.3 ounces	76 milligrams
Coffee, home brewed	8 ounces	65 to 120 milligrams
Mountain Dew	12 ounces	55 milligrams
Tea	8 ounces	40 to 120 milligrams
Cola	12 ounces	35 milligrams
Sprite	12 ounces	0 milligram
Medications:		
NoDoz, maximum strength	1 tablet	200 milligrams
Excedrin, extra strength	2 tablets	160 milligrams
Anacin, maximum strength	2 tablets	64 milligrams

Source: starbucks.com, package labels, mayoclinic.com

How Much Is Too Much?

Tolerance or sensitivity to caffeine varies from person to person. But a moderate amount of caffeine is 300 milligrams per day, or about 2 cups of mild coffee.

In addition to increasing the movement in your intestines, which may trigger pain and/or diarrhea, being overcaffeinated can make you irritable and jittery and contribute to headaches. Listening to your body and having a greater awareness of your caffeine intake helps you adjust your intake as necessary.

Slowing down, taking time to chew, and managing portions is a good part of your healthy lifestyle. Keep it real with the caffeine and alcohol, and you'll be well on your way to keeping your body happy.

The Least You Need to Know

- ◆ Digestion begins in your mouth, so slow down when you eat and chew thoroughly for your best digestion.

- ◆ Replace large meals with smaller, more frequent ones. Grazing is best for IBS.

- ◆ Avoid straws, carbonated beverages, and gum, and you avoid extra air intake, which contributes to gas and bloating.

- ◆ Moderation is key when consuming alcohol and caffeine. Know your limits!

Probiotics: Digestive Helpers

In This Chapter

◆ Gut bacteria: it's good for you!

◆ How gut bacteria help your immune system

◆ Probiotics: an IBS cure-all?

◆ The down side of prebiotics

Have you ever heard the saying, "You've got to eat a peck of dirt before you die"? You might think that sounds, well, less than appetizing, but the reality is, a bit of dirt in your food can do the body good. Okay, not *dirt* per se, but how does bacteria sound? When it comes right down to it, our bodies reap hefty benefits from consuming friendly bacteria found in cultured food such as yogurt, fermented foods, or in supplements. The bacteria that provide the body with the most health benefits are known as *probiotics*. More and more scientific studies are linking probiotics to potential improvement in symptoms for those with IBS.

Although we've adopted a cleaner-is-better philosophy, with antibacterial products in our soaps and cleaners, we likely need a bit more bacteria in our food. Let's learn more about probiotics and their potential role in IBS symptom management. You may find you need a few more microbes in your life!

Good-for-You Gut Bacteria

You have about 2 or 3 pounds of bugs living primarily in your intestines. Sounds like something you'd see in a creepy sci-fi movie, right? Well, this is real. The bacteria in your intestines are known as *intestinal flora*, and you have more than 400 different types of them in there. The flora contains good and bad bacteria. Maintaining proper balance between the two appears to be key for good health. Adding healthy bacteria such as probiotics to your diet is a good way to preserve intestinal bacterial balance.

Wellness Words _____

Probiotics are bacteria that provide positive health benefits to the body. *Probiotic* stands for "pro-life." **Intestinal flora** are the bacteria that normally reside in your intestines.

According to the World Health Organization, probiotics are "live microorganisms which when administered in adequate amounts confer a health benefit on the host." According to the National Center for Complementary and Alternative Medicine, interest in probiotics is up lately, as Americans spent nearly triple the amount on probiotics in 2003 compared to 1994.

In some cases, such as those with an immature or weakened immune system, probiotics may be harmful and can actually contribute to infection. For this reason, before introducing supplements into your IBS management plan, be sure to discuss the appropriateness of their use in your body with your doctor.

What Science Tells Us About Probiotics

The role of probiotics in health and intestinal well-being is still being researched, and experts don't have a full understanding of how supplemental probiotics operate in the human body. Because of this, general guidelines for their use are limited. We do know that intestinal bacteria play an important role in nutritional health because they help produce vitamin K and folate. Vitamin K plays an essential role in blood clotting, while folate helps produce and maintain cells. Probiotics also help with degradation of food, aiding digestion. New evidence links gut bacteria to enhanced immune function and a possible role in autoimmune disease prevention.

Studying the effectiveness of probiotics in human health is difficult because there are many different species and strains of bacteria. Research has shown that different probiotic strains—even if they're from the same species—can exert different effects on the body. Scientists still need more well-designed studies to be able to make general recommendations for specific species, strains, amounts, and timing of probiotic use.

Of all the many studies evaluating probiotic use and IBS, the most compelling involves Bifidobacterium infantis 35264. Studies reviewing the impact of bifidobacterium in IBS suffers have shown a reduction in pain and gas while enhancing well-being. Other strains of bifidobacterium have proven helpful in regulating constipation by increasing stool frequency after three weeks of product consumption.

In addition, a number of studies have been performed to evaluate the effectiveness of supplemental probiotics and various health conditions. The most convincing studies to date reveal such benefits as:

◆ A decrease in antibiotic-induced diarrhea

◆ A lessening in the duration of the diarrhea phase of rotavirus infection

◆ A decrease in diarrhea, pain, and bloating in those with IBS, particularly with bifidobacteria

According to 2008's *An Evidence-Based Systematic Review on the Management of Irritable Bowel Syndrome* by the American College of Gastroenterology, probiotic use of single organisms of lactobacilli do not appear to be effective in management of IBS. But bifidobacteria and certain combinations of probiotics did show some usefulness in treating IBS management by improving symptoms and quality of life measures. There may be some type of synergistic effect, meaning that bacteria work together, in IBS management. For this reason, it may be beneficial to include a variety of probiotics in your diet versus sticking with just one source. This is easy to do with yogurt that contains live and active cultures, as many brands include a variety of bacteria cultures.

Gut Facts

Not all bacteria or cultured food contain probiotics. In order for bacteria to be labeled a probiotic, it must exert positive health benefits.

More Friendly Bacteria You Should Know

The two most commonly known families of friendly bugs are *lactobacillus* and *bifidobacteria*. Both can be consumed in food or found in supplement form. The best-known probiotic is lactobacillus acidophilus, which is found commonly in yogurt. Studies evaluating lactobacillus continue to emerge and show some potential in helping the body absorb nutrients, preventing overgrowth of the unfriendly bacteria, averting urinary infections, and decreasing duration of the diarrhea phase of rotavirus infection.

> **Wellness Words** _____
>
> **Lactobacillus** is a category of bacteria considered beneficial to the human body. **Bifidobacteria** is a healthful bacteria or probiotic that shows the most benefit for managing IBS symptoms.

Bifidobacteria, found in breast milk and in many yogurts, plays a role in regulating movement of the intestine, known as peristalsis. Bifidobacteria and lactobaccillus help produce an acid environment in the intestine, which has been speculated to decrease or prevent the growth of some yeast and other unhealthy bacteria.

Maintaining Gut Balance

Maintaining intestinal balance can be tricky for the person with IBS because undigested foods provide a constant supply of nutrients for the intestinal flora, allowing them to flourish. Medications can impact gut balance, too, as antibiotics, steroids, and antacids kill off friendly bacteria, allowing yeasts and bad bacteria to grow out of control.

Because the person with IBS has alterations in digestion ranging from an overactive intestine to a sluggish bowel, gut bacteria can be impacted. When certain bacteria overgrow, this imbalance can set off your IBS symptoms. Small intestinal bacterial overgrowth, as reviewed in Chapter 1, is an example of intestinal flora being out of balance. Too many bacteria infiltrating the small bowel lead to gas, bloating, and other IBS symptoms. It's not a pretty picture, is it?

Introducing Dysbiosis

Dysbiosis is another one of the crazy medical terms I enjoy throwing your way. (I sometimes wonder who creates some of these medical terms!) Dysbiosis refers to an imbalance in intestinal bacteria. Causes of dysbiosis include overuse of antibiotics, antacids, and processed foods, and also malabsorption.

The antibiotics you use to kill the bacteria causing an infection in your body can also kill off the healthful bacteria in your intestine. And remember from earlier chapters that malabsorption means the food you're eating is making its way to your large intestine and providing excess food for bacteria to eat. All this helps create an imbalance of gut bacteria.

Replenish Your Supply

Because your bacteria supply can be affected by medication use and the way your body absorbs foods—or should I say, lack of absorption of food with IBS—replenishing your gut bacteria might require some work on your part and will likely prove beneficial for your symptom control.

As noted earlier, probiotics are found in foods and in supplement form. You can find capsules, powders, and dairy-infused supplements at many grocery stores and pharmacies. Yogurt, kefir, miso, and tempeh can contain probiotics, which may have been added or present during the manufacturing of the product, so consider giving these a try, too.

Here are some other simple ways to incorporate probiotics in your diet:

◆ Eat cultured yogurt made with "live and active cultures."

◆ Look for yogurt that offers a variety of different strains of bacteria.

◆ Try lassi, a cultured Indian beverage.

◆ Culturelle (lactobacillus) and Align (bifidobacteria) are commercially available probiotics with a number of scientific studies revealing various health benefits.

Supplements and Food Sources

The view that cultured foods are healthful has been recognized for many years. In countries outside the United States, cultured foods are customary. In Asia, fermented soy sauce is a staple. In European households, sauerkraut (a fermented form of cabbage) is eaten regularly. I was recently introduced to lassi, a drink enjoyed frequently in India. Lassi is a fermented dairy drink, a cool yogurt smoothie of sorts that comes in a salty or sweet version. It's very refreshing.

Gut Facts

The National Center for Complementary and Alternative Medicine (NCCAM) is one of the 27 institutes or centers that make up the National Institutes of Health. NCCAM is a great resource for alternative medicine and probiotic therapy. Check out nccam.nih.gov/health for more information.

In America, food manufacturers are catching on, as the value of probiotics is being scientifically documented. More and more food products supplemented with these healthful bugs can be found in supermarkets—and probably a grocer near you!

Increasing healthful bacteria is quite easy to do. In fact, you really don't need any specialized products; regular yogurt will often do the trick. But read on to learn about what you need to know to pick the best cultured foods for you.

If consuming probiotics via yogurt, be sure the yogurt label states that it contains live and active cultures. Even if the product is made with live and active cultures, it may *not* contain live cultures after it's been pasteurized. Additionally, many supplements are best kept in the refrigerator because the cool temperature keeps the bacteria alive while others are specially designed to not require refrigeration. Be sure to store probiotics as noted on their label.

If you're particularly sensitive to dairy sources, which are the more common probiotic-rich food in the United States, consider a supplement such as Align, which contains bifidobacteria. Sometimes when my intestines are particularly out of whack, I prefer limiting my lactose completely and opt for this supplement. It really helps me get back in balance. (Yes, I do practice what I preach!)

Prebiotics: Good or Bad?

Prebiotics are undigested food that provides nourishment for the *probiotics* residing in your large intestine. Like any other living being, when there's food available, the intestinal bacteria grow and thrive.

Two of the more commonly known prebiotics are inulin and fructooligosaccharides, or FOS, which you might remember from Chapter 2. These prebiotics are part of the oligosaccharide family (they are the *O* in the acronym FODMAP). For the person with IBS, these prebiotics can contribute to IBS symptoms. Remember, IBS bodies are prone to digestion issues, so adding more indigestible components to the mix can be problematic. FOS and inulin are often added to products as a way to boost the fiber, lower the fat, or modify the sugar content of food products.

Wellness Words

Prebiotics are nondigestible food sources that selectively feed intestinal bacteria.

Both inulin and FOS stimulate the growth of bifidobacteria, a well-known healthy bacteria. Neither one is absorbed by the human body, so they don't stimulate insulin release or increase blood sugar. This is an appealing feature to food manufacturers because FOS and inulin make a better carbohydrate source for food products marketed to diabetics. Both inulin and FOS are used worldwide as a fiber source in foods.

Inulin

Inulin is widely found in nature as a plant's storage form of carbohydrates. Inulin is made up of long chains of the molecule fructose. Common sources of inulin include wheat, onions, asparagus, garlic, and chicory root.

Inulin has been used to replace fat in foods, too. Some probiotic supplements have added inulin as a prebiotic. Because inulin can lead to IBS symptoms, if choosing a probiotic-rich food or supplement, you may want to choose one that does not contain inulin.

> **Gut Facts**
>
> You probably think you've never had chicory root, but think again. Chicory root extract is used commonly as an added fiber ingredient in many everyday products and supplements, including yogurt, spreads, and baked goods.

FOS

FOS is sometimes referred to as oligofructose or oligofructan. FOS is similar in structure to inulin but typically contains a smaller chain of fructose molecules. It also tends to be more soluble or able to mix with water than inulin. For this reason, FOS is more desirable in dairy products, frozen desserts, and some bakery goods. FOS makes cookies crispier. Both FOS and inulin are added to foods to provide fiber and for their role as probiotic food.

Because FOS is a FODMAP family member, it may be problematic in the IBS sufferer.

When it comes to probiotic use and IBS, most experts agree that there's promising evidence probiotics are helpful in symptom management. Bifidobacterium infantis 35624 marketed commercially as Align has shown the most promise in IBS management.

The intestine is an important part of the immune system, and it's been proposed that keeping gut bacteria in proper balance enhances your ability to fight infection as well as enhance the immune function. Studies continue to emerge in this important area of gastrointestinal health, so be sure to keep an eye on the science by visiting www.pubmed.gov. It's always good to stay on top of any new research in IBS treatment to help you best manage your health.

The Least You Need to Know

- Research is starting to support the use of probiotics in managing IBS.

- Bifidobacterium infantis 35264 has been shown to be most effective in IBS management.

- Probiotics have been shown to help minimize antibiotic-induced diarrhea.

- Prebiotics provide food for the probiotic bacteria to grow and flourish in your intestine. Some prebiotics, such as inulin and FOS, can be IBS triggers.

Part 2

Smart Strategies for IBS-Free Living

Now that you know all about your IBS body and its triggers, you can apply what you've learned to living your best, pain-free life. Making smart food choices can be a daunting task while grocery shopping and when dining out or away from home. Because life can be busy, you need a few tools to make living in the real world a bit easier.

Part 2 covers everything you need to know about making healthful meals, identifying the best choices at restaurants, and creating a travel survival kit. I walk you through the grocery store with a healthful shopping list in hand, help you become the best dining-out detective, and prepare you for easier traveling, all while keeping your IBS on the right path.

Chapter 7

Grocery Shopping and Menu Planning

In This Chapter

- Good menu planning = healthy eating
- Curbing impulse buying
- Learning to choose the best foods
- Finding your best-tolerated foods
- Menu suggestions to get you started

Now is the time to put together all you've learned about foods and your IBS symptoms in Part 1 and start bringing home the best foods for your body. What you have at home is usually what you eat, so be sure to have the right foods on hand. Choosing wholesome, nourishing foods helps manage your IBS symptoms, but also likely improves your health as well!

In this chapter, we walk through the grocery store and learn some key tips on selecting the best foods for your IBS body. Strategic menu planning ensures that you purchase all the necessary ingredients for new and nourishing recipes you might want to try. With smart menu planning, you guarantee less impulse pizza delivery or fast-food meals, which we know are not the best food choices for your irritable bowel.

Navigating the Grocery Store

With the advent of the mega- and super-grocery stores, it's a wonder you can find what you're looking for when you shop for food. You can get furniture in aisle one, tuna in aisle two, and your shoes shined in aisle three! You need a GPS just to pick up a few fresh dinner ingredients!

Here's a great tip for navigating most markets: sticking to the outer walls of most grocery stores keeps you where you want to be, with the freshest and best-for-you foods. Don't get hung up in the middle where all the other stuff is.

Shop Smart

Your first stop in the grocery store should be the produce section. Here, fill up on your favorite produce (or what you can tolerate). Here are some good low-FODMAP choices to consider adding to your cart, again, based on what you can tolerate:

- Bell peppers
- Blueberries
- Carrots
- Grape tomatoes
- Kiwifruit

- Lettuce
- Mushrooms
- Oranges
- Squash
- Strawberries

When making your selections, think color! Try to pick something red, orange, blue/purple, white, and green. In general, the brighter the produce, the more nutritious it is for you.

Digestibles _____

Check out the Centers for Disease Control's website at www.fruitsandveggiesmatter. gov to learn more about how many fruits and vegetables you should be consuming based on your age and sex. With lots of great fruit and vegetable recipes and tips to increase your intake, you'll soon be the healthiest person on the block!

Next, off to the meat counter. Here, choose lean cuts of beef such as London broil, flank steak, and tenderloin to go easy on your fat intake. Your best pork cuts include tenderloin and center-cut chops. Boneless chicken, ground chicken, turkey tenderloin, and ground turkey breast make great poultry picks. To change it up a bit, try some turkey bacon or chicken sausage. (These are lower in fat content but not always lower in sodium, so don't rely on these completely.) Fish is also a lean and terrific protein selection.

In the dairy aisle, look for low-fat choices such as skim or 1 percent milk rather than full-fat whole milk. If lactose is a problem for you, choose reduced-lactose milk and reduced-lactose cottage cheese. Choose the hard cheeses such as cheddar, Parmesan, and Swiss for lower-lactose alternatives. Here's where you can find rice "cheese" as well. Probiotics-rich yogurt is a great option, too. Try Greek-style yogurt for a rich protein source.

While spinning through the bread section, choose whole-grain choices that come in smaller portion sizes such as whole-wheat English muffins instead of huge bagels, or sandwich bread versus large rolls. This helps minimize your wheat intake, which can be helpful when dealing with IBS.

Closer to Nature

Follow my train of thought here a minute. The store's inside aisles most often contain convenience packaged foods, salad dressings, canned soups, boxed crackers, candy, and snacks. Now think about what's along the outside perimeter of the store—produce, fresh breads and grains, fresh meat and seafood, etc. There's little to no processed foods here!

One of your food-shopping goals should be to buy foods that already exist in nature, or are as close to their natural state as you can find. Think of foods you'd find on a local farm or in a backyard garden. Consuming food in its natural form versus processed is a good start for eating a wholesome diet. Face it, chocolate cream–filled cakes do not grow on trees!

Tummy Trouble _____

The end caps on most aisles host the specials of the week, such as buy 10 for $10, buy one get one free, etc. At these prices, you almost feel the store is paying you to buy the product! Stop for a moment, and ask yourself if you really need that food. Is it a healthy choice for your family? Make the right decision, and don't let the deal of the day influence you.

Minimize Processed Foods

If most of your meal-planning instructions include "just add water and serve," you're likely filling up on processed foods. The problem with processed foods is that they're often loaded with additives, preservatives, extra salt, artificial colors, and who knows what else.

Your body doesn't crave preservatives or red dye #3, and it sure doesn't need partially hydrogenated fats and high-fructose corn syrup (HFCS) that lurk in many of these "quick-fix" meals. If you must, choose these foods in a pinch, but certainly don't make them a regular part of your menu plan.

How Smart Is Your Cart?

Have you ever looked at the grocery carts around you in the supermarket and realized how unhealthfully some people eat (maybe you included!)? I walk around my local grocery store feeling like the queen of health—or sometimes like I have the baddest-looking cart in town!

Keeping your cart smart involves two key ingredients: making sure you shop on a full stomach and arriving with a well-planned grocery list.

Making a List and Checking It Twice

Using a checklist helps you get what you need at the grocery store—and nothing you don't need. Here's a sample list you can copy and take with you—or use as inspiration when you make your own:

Fruit—fresh or frozen without extra ingredients are best:

- ❏ Bananas
- ❏ Blueberries
- ❏ Grapefruit
- ❏ Kiwifruit
- ❏ Lemons
- ❏ Limes
- ❏ Oranges

❏ Strawberries

❏ Tomatoes

Vegetables—fresh or frozen without added ingredients are best:

❏ Beets

❏ Broccoli

❏ Carrots

❏ Celery

❏ Corn

❏ Cucumbers

❏ Eggplants

❏ Fresh herbs—basil, parsley

❏ Green beans

❏ Green peas

❏ Lettuce

❏ Potatoes

❏ Snow peas

❏ Spinach

❏ Summer squash

❏ Sweet bell peppers

❏ Sweet potatoes

❏ Turnips

❏ Winter squash

Grain products:

❏ Corn tortillas

❏ Oat-based cold cereals

❏ Old-fashioned oats

❑ Pasta—rice, corn, wheat

❑ Rice—brown, forbidden, whole-grain

❑ Steel-cut oats

❑ Whole-grain breads, bagels, English muffins

Canned/jar products:

❑ Peanut butter, all natural

❑ Reduced-fat and -sodium broth

❑ Tomatoes—diced, crushed

❑ Tuna

Dairy products:

❑ Butter—try spreadable forms mixed with oils

❑ Egg substitute

❑ Eggs

❑ Greek-style yogurt—vanilla, plain

❑ Milk—skim, 1 percent

❑ Naturally low-lactose cheese—Swiss, cheddar, Parmesan

❑ Reduced-fat cheese

❑ Reduced-lactose low-fat cottage cheese

❑ Reduced-lactose low-fat milk

❑ Traditional yogurt—vanilla, plain

❑ Trans fat–free tub margarine

Meats:

❑ Beef—lean cuts such as London broil, flank, top round, sirloin

❑ Chicken—boneless, skinless, ground chicken breast

❑ Ham

❏ Pork—center-cut chop, tenderloin

❏ Turkey—breast, tenderloin, ground turkey breast

Seafood:

❏ Fish

❏ Shellfish—all types

Baking ingredients:

❏ Baking powder

❏ Baking soda

❏ Cocoa

❏ Corn starch

❏ Extracts—vanilla, coconut, almond

❏ Flour—wheat, white rice, brown rice

❏ Garlic powder

❏ Nuts—unsalted walnuts, almonds, and peanuts

❏ Oils—canola, olive

❏ Spices—basil, garlic powder, Italian seasoning, thyme, and onion powder

❏ Sugar—brown, granulated, confectioners'

Snack foods:

❏ Baked potato chips

❏ Corn cakes

❏ Crackers—rice, nut, whole grain

❏ Granola bars

❏ Popcorn

❏ Rice cakes

❏ Tortilla chips

Creating a thorough list of all the foods you need for the week is a good start to strategic shopping. Be sure to include all the ingredients for new recipes you plan on trying, too. Avoid shopping without a list because it's too easy to get distracted and buy on impulse.

Creating Menu Plans with Your Grocery List

It's easy to coordinate your menu planning and grocery list. All you need is an 8½×11 sheet of paper and a pen or pencil (or the computer equivalents if you prefer). On the left side of the sheet, list your menus. On the right side, list the grocery items you'll need for those menus, including anything for the new recipes you plan on trying.

When you're done shopping, save the list as a reminder of the menu plans you put together for the week. This keeps you better focused with your meal planning and shopping than you can imagine—give it a try!

IBS-Friendly Meal Planning

So how do you put all this nutrition information into practice? Start planning some IBS-friendly menus by incorporating what you've learned from filling in your food diary (see Chapter 4 for more on your food diary). Then flip to Part 3 in this book and look over the recipes I've included there. Starting with breakfast, pick some recipes to try. Shoot for trying one new recipe a week. When planning lunch menus, select brown bag–friendly recipes or try leftovers from dinner the night before.

Remember, a balanced plate provides your body with good nutrition and the proper balance it needs.

Gut Facts _____

Frozen vegetables with no added fats or salt offer similar nutritional content when compared to fresh produce—and often cost less! Because most produce has traveled miles to arrive at your local store, it's been exposed to light and heat, which reduce its nutritional value. Fresh and locally grown produce give you the biggest payout when it comes to preserved nutrition, but when local seasonal produce isn't available, give the frozen version a try.

Breaking the Nighttime Fast: Breakfast

Don't skip this important meal of the day! Begin your day on the right foot with some nourishing goodness. A bit of whole grains and protein paired with a fruit or vegetable will set you up for your day. Here are some suggestions to help you break the fast:

- Whole-grain English muffin with peanut butter and an orange

- Creamy Slow Cooker Oatmeal (recipe in Chapter 11) with cranberries, almonds, and maple syrup with a cup of low-fat vanilla yogurt

- Ham and Rosemary Omelet (recipe in Chapter 10) with two slices of brown rice bread, toasted, and some fresh strawberries

- Almond-Vanilla-Blueberry Parfait (recipe in Chapter 12)

- Cold oat–based cereal with lactaid milk and a small, ripe banana

If you find it hard to eat first thing in the morning, fix a breakfast to take with you. You may find you could use a little nourishment mid-morning. No one says you have to eat immediately upon arising!

Midday Break: Lunch

Depending on where you typically eat lunch, at home where you can cook up a lavish meal or at work where you have to grab a quick bite, you can adjust your expectations and menu-planning depending on what works best for you and your schedule. Here are some lunch-worthy suggestions:

- Brown rice or corn tortilla filled with brown rice, shredded chicken, grated cheddar cheese, tomatoes, and chopped lettuce with some baby carrots and a cup of blueberries

- Pita pocket filled with tuna salad, lettuce, and tomatoes with some sugar snap peas (these are delicious raw), a small ripe banana, and a handful of almonds

- A bowl of Grandma's Chicken and Rice soup (recipe in Chapter 14) with a kiwifruit and a handful of rice crackers or nut crackers

- Farmer's Market Pasta Salad (recipe in Chapter 18) with a side of grilled shrimp and an orange.

What's for Dinner?

As a mom of three, there are nights when shuffling around my kitchen is simply not an option due to sports games or work commitments. On these nights, I opt for a slow cooker meal or allow for some healthful take-out food.

I enjoy cooking, so when I have the time, I often make a brown rice or wheat pasta salad in advance and serve that for lunch and dinner throughout the week. With teenage boys, having food ready to roll makes my life easier. Grabbing a rotisserie chicken, microwavable frozen vegetables, and brown rice, I can have dinner on the table in six minutes flat. In that short time, you'll be eating dinner sooner than any pizza guy could deliver.

Here are some great dinner fixes for you, your family, and your sensitive intestines:

♦ Grilled chicken, rice pasta, peas, and a garden salad

♦ Flank steak, broccoli (tolerance varies for broccoli, so limit if it troubles you), and a baked potato

♦ Sautéed shrimp, brown rice, and sliced carrots

♦ Asian Chicken Lettuce Wraps (recipe in Chapter 17) with brown rice sautéed with mushrooms and peas

♦ Center-Cut Chops with Dijon (recipe in Chapter 17), Sweet Potato Fries (recipe in Chapter 19), and a spinach salad

For the In-Between Times: Snacks

Because smaller, more frequent meals are best tolerated in IBS, being a good snacker is a requirement. If your lifestyle warrants that you're away from a refrigerator during the day, pack granola bars, an oat-based cereal you can put in a zipper-lock bag, $\frac{1}{4}$ cup nuts, or an orange to take with you on your way out the door. If you can, stop and make a smoothie or a parfait (see Chapter 12 for great options). I love smoothies as a quick snack, and they're a great source of protein, probiotics, and just enough fruit.

Snacks should be a mini meal, just enough to keep you satisfied, not a full-meal-size portion. If you start eating six full meals a day, you soon may have to contend with a weight issue!

Here are some power-packed snacks to try:

◆ Fruit smoothies (recipes in Chapter 12)

◆ Chunk of reduced-fat cheddar cheese with nut or rice crackers

◆ ½ whole-wheat English muffin with peanut butter

◆ Oat-based granola bar (Avoid those with high-fructose corn syrup or inulin.)

◆ ½ cup yogurt with 2 tablespoons granola and 2 tablespoons strawberries or blueberries

◆ 6 to 8 whole-grain crackers with ¼ cup reduced-lactose cottage cheese

Digestibles

Purchase frozen mixed berries and store in your freezer for quick-fix smoothies or defrost a cup in a bowl in your refrigerator before you go to bed. When you wake up, toss the defrosted berries and syrup over your plain or vanilla yogurt. Yum!

Healthful eating requires good planning. Your health is in your hands, so take a few minutes each week and put together a list of menus and required grocery items. In the long run, you'll not only feel better, you'll also save time, money, and aggravation!

Having enjoyable meals your body can tolerate will make a world of difference in your quality of life. My 84-year-old mom says, "A stitch in time saves nine." In a sense, the same is true in IBS. If you take the time to purchase and prepare the right foods for your IBS body, you save countless days trying to get your tummy back on track.

The Least You Need to Know

◆ By shopping the perimeter of the grocery store, you'll find the most wholesome food choices, similar to those found in nature. The less processed the food, the more likely it will offer greater nutritional value.

◆ By shopping with a detailed grocery list and menu options for the week, you'll eat healthier and minimize impulse pizza deliveries or drive-thru fast-food dinners.

◆ Having healthful foods at home encourages healthier eating. What you bring into the house is what you eat, so bring home nourishing foods.

◆ Your best bets are brightly colored produce selections, low-fat meats and fish, low-lactose and low-fat dairy choices, and whole grains and nuts.

Chapter 8

Dining Out Without Consequence

In This Chapter

- ◆ Serving size versus portion size
- ◆ Tips for controlling portions
- ◆ Choosing IBS-friendly drinks
- ◆ Getting what you need when eating out

I probably don't have to tell you restaurant portion sizes have morphed from reasonable to gargantuan over the past couple decades. It's difficult to leave a restaurant these days without feeling stuffed to the gills. Unlimited tortilla chips, baskets of bread, and 20-ounce drinks even before your large meal arrives served on a huge platter all contribute to overeating.

In this chapter, I reveal appropriate portion size for your IBS body, along with great strategies for choosing your best beverages and entrées while still enjoying your dining-out experience. Learning how to ask specifically for what you need and how foods are prepared can be your best tool when eating away from home.

Keeping Portion Sizes Real

Understanding portion sizes can be a bit complicated. *Portion size* and *serving size* are often used interchangeably, but they definitely don't mean the same thing. A serving size reflects the amount of food listed on the nutrition facts label, while portion size refers to how much of the food you should eat at a meal or snack time.

Foods are often grouped in serving sizes depicting a similar amount of calories or nutritional component. For instance, a 1-ounce piece of bread, ⅓ cup of rice, and ½ cup of pasta all have about 80 calories and 15 grams of carbohydrates. These are often grouped together as serving sizes of starches or carbohydrates.

Unless you're 3 years old, you likely eat a bit more than ⅓ cup of rice at a sitting, right? The serving size may be ⅓ cup, while the portion size for most people should be 1 cup. Ever get take-out Chinese food? Check out the rice portion. At about 5 cups, that would translate to 15 serving sizes, or about 5 portion sizes.

Digestibles

Fruit serving sizes are a good tool to help you minimize fructose in your diet. Limit fruit to one serving size per meal or snack time. That could mean ½ cup chopped fruit, ½ large banana, 15 to 18 grapes, ¾ cup blueberries, 1 small orange, or 1 cup strawberries.

Sometimes serving size and portion size equate to the same amount of food. For example, 6 to 8 crackers, the serving size, is an appropriate portion for your snack.

When looking at the nutrition facts label, it's easy to feel like you're overdoing your portions because the serving sizes are comparatively small. I think, however, the serving size is a reliable gauge when eating a between-meal snack.

Keep It in Balance

When eating meals, learning how to balance your plate for best portion control is critical. If you imagine your plate divided into sections, half of it should be filled with colorful, tolerated vegetables. One fourth should contain a lean protein source. The other fourth should be filled with a starchy food such as rice, potato, bread, peas, pasta, millet, kasha, or other tolerable grains.

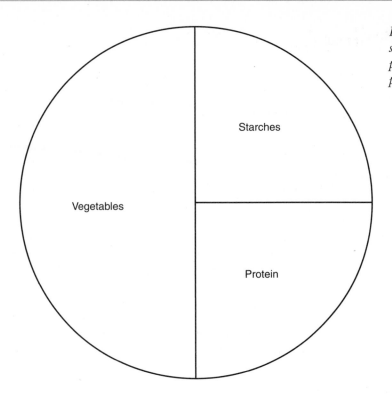

Balancing the vegetables, starches, and protein on your plate is important for good portion control.

Here are some great lean protein sources to add to your plate:

◆ Fish or shellfish

◆ Skinless chicken or turkey breast, ground turkey breast, or ground chicken breast

◆ Beef tenderloin, London broil, flank steak, beef round, or >90-percent-lean beef burger

◆ Pork tenderloin, center-cut chops, center loin, or Canadian bacon

Typically, restaurants load up your plate with larger meats and starchy food portions with few to no vegetables. That leads to an unbalanced plate, and an unbalanced plate leads to an unbalanced you!

Mindless Versus Mindful Eating

Numerous studies have shown that when people are offered larger servings, they eat more. It's often as simple as that. If it's there, you'll eat it. In his book *Mindless Eating: Why We Eat More Than We Think* (Hay House, 2009), researcher Brian Wansink provides many studies revealing how many of us mindlessly overeat at restaurants.

Do you eat mindlessly? Eating mindlessly means you're not conscious of eating. Eating while on the computer, while watching television, or anytime your mind is elsewhere are examples of eating mindlessly. When you're eating and aren't cognizant of the eating process, you may even forget to chew your foods properly. You may easily overeat because you're not necessarily paying attention. Have you ever found yourself eating a snack food from a bag or box and find your hand hitting the bottom of the container, leaving you incredulous that you actually ate that much? That happens to me at the movie theater. The popcorn seems to go so quickly when I'm busy watching the movie!

When you don't clue in to the taste and aroma of the foods you eat, you may not derive as much pleasure from the food. Why? Because you're thinking about other things! Notice how great food can taste when you pay attention. Try *mindfully* eating a piece of chocolate. Take a small square of chocolate, place it in your mouth, and slowly let it melt. Feel the texture, and breathe in the aroma. This is a great way to eat with IBS. When you eat foods this way, you'll likely enjoy them more and eat less.

Eating mindfully offers even more health benefits. For one, you digest foods better and likely eat less, helping with weight management. It takes about 20 minutes for your stomach to let your brain know it's full. When you eat mindfully and methodically, your brain will likely get the message before you have a chance to overeat.

Recommended Versus Real Portions

Package labels often don't depict what most average people should and often do eat, so work on balancing your plate as your first-line strategy for keeping portions reasonable and realistic. When dining out, ordering a baked potato and two sides of vegetables helps you get closer to your ideal meal. A large pasta portion, with a shred of vegetables and meat, however, is not a well-balanced meal.

If you do choose a pasta- or pizza-based meal, order a salad first to load up on your veggies while filling your belly. When meal portions are over the top, plan on sharing the meal or bringing home half of the meal in a doggie bag. You could even ask the server to pack half your order in a to-go container and bring the other half to the table. That way, you're not even tempted to eat more than you should.

Check out the following table to help visualize reasonable portions of some common foods.

Food	Size of Reasonable Portion
1 cup cereal	1 fist
1 cup pasta or mashed potatoes	1 baseball
1 baked potato	1 fist
2 tablespoons peanut butter	1 ping-pong ball
1½ ounces cheese	4 stacked dice

Source: National Institutes of Health

Tips to Curb Your Intake

A few tricks can help you manage your portions. I've learned that overeating at restaurants is a sure way to trigger my IBS. My husband and I often share an entrée or an appetizer, and this makes a world of difference. Avoiding restaurants that offer huge portions or buffets where overindulging is almost inevitable is a good start to keep you away from temptation.

Here are a few more tips to help you and your intestines stay on track:

◆ Don't skip meals in anticipation of dining out; that can lead to overeating.

◆ Fill up on soup or salad first.

◆ Split an entrée and either a dessert or an appetizer—not both!

◆ Eat slowly, putting your fork down between bites.

◆ Say no to extra free rolls or tortilla chips.

◆ Remember, this is not the last supper. You'll have other opportunities to have these favorite foods again. So go easy now.

 Tummy Trouble

Munching a couple rolls prior to your meal adds fructans to your diet, which can aggravate your IBS and add about 300 extra calories to your meal. Skip the bread!

It took me a while to realize that when dining out, I didn't have to leave the restaurant uncomfortably full. When I was a little girl, my father loved taking our family to different restaurants. One of his favorites in Boston offered popovers and cheese with crackers, before our meal even came to the table. I can vividly remembering unbuckling my belt on the ride home after feasting on the popovers and my dinner!

A good meal should never leave you feeling sick. Your body is very efficient at talking back to you when things aren't working; be sure to listen to it!

Think Before You Drink

Is that a beverage glass or a trough you are drinking from? I always find it amazing at some restaurants when drink glasses come out from the bar. Some drink sizes are seriously over the top! Have you noticed these same types of restaurants offer free refills? This can be a big-time problem for the IBS sufferer. Soft drinks, lemonade, and iced tea often contain large quantities of high-fructose corn syrup (HFCS), as well as caffeine, which can be an issue in IBS. (Remember the whole excess fructose–IBS connection.) And that's even before you factor in all the carbonation!

Choose your drink as if your intestinal health depended on it … because it does! If you don't, you may find the payback is more than you bargained for. Your best bet: choose water! A small glass of orange juice, soft drink, seltzer, club soda with a bit of cranberry and a lime, or wine should be tolerated just fine. Did I say *small* glass? Yes. Stick with a *small* glass when it comes to beverages to control your intake of carbonation and HFCS. If you're ready for a second drink, go for a glass of water.

Again with the Portion Sizes

Looking at drink portions more closely, you can see why size does matter. It's not uncommon in my private practice to find a number of clients who have gained unnecessary weight—not from what they're eating, but what they're drinking on a regular basis. Studies have shown that those who consume sugar-filled drinks don't appear to compensate by reducing calorie intake in foods, so they tend to gain weight.

Take a peek at some of the offensive numbers shown in the following table.

What's in Your Drink?

Beverage	Amount	Calories	Sugar
Orange juice	20 ounces	300	19 teaspoons
Hot chocolate (2% milk)	20 ounces	370	15 teaspoons
Soft drink	20 ounces	250	17 teaspoons
Sweetened iced tea	20 ounces	175	11 teaspoons
Unsweetened tea or coffee	20 ounces	0	0 teaspoon
Water	20 ounces	0	0 teaspoon

Many restaurants serve 20-ounce portions with free refills, even if you don't ask! Don't be tempted to fill and refill—or drink the refills your server keeps bringing. You'll end up with too many calories and too much sugar if you do, which you'll probably pay for later.

Liquid Assets

With IBS, choosing your best beverages involves more than calorie control, as some beverages contain ingredients that are irritants for the IBS body. For instance, HFCS found readily in soft drinks can be problematic in large quantities. Remember, the human body can only absorb so much extra fructose. Carbonation can also be a problem. Beer made with wheat ingredients can be troublesome, too. Alcohol and caffeine in moderation may or may not be tolerated, so keep a check on your symptoms using your food diary from Chapter 4.

Concerned about what your drink might contain that could trigger your IBS? Check out the following table for some common beverage choices and potential problem areas.

Beware Beverage Choices

Beverage	Concerns
Beer	Wheat, carbonation, alcohol
Cappuccino/latte	Lactose, caffeine
Juice	Portion size/fructose

continues

Beware Beverage Choices (continued)

Beverage	Concerns
Soft drinks	HFCS, carbonation, caffeine (some)
Water	None
Wine	Alcohol
Wine spritzer	Alcohol, carbonation

Another alternative is to try smaller portions of your favorite beverages (ask the server for a kid's size portion) or opt for a small club soda with just a splash of juice. Order cappuccino with soy milk, or order one "dry," which uses much less milk and therefore less lactose, and more foam. That works for me! Choosing decaf coffee drinks is another option if caffeine is a trigger for you.

Your Mind-Set Matters

If you've not picked up on my not-so-subtle hints yet, let me spell it out for you: you have to think about what you eat and drink and how it'll affect your IBS. Especially when dining out, you need a strategic plan. To execute your strategy effectively, you need to go into the restaurant with a game plan. Don't allow impulse choices or swaying from friends or family to get you off your healthful IBS path.

Knowing whether you intend to indulge in an appetizer, desserts, and a certain number of beverages is a good pre–dining out plan. It's usually the impulsive decisions that cause the most grief. Many restaurants offer menus online or in the window. Take a peek at them prior to dining out to get your game plan set up. Be sure IBS-friendly meals are available. If not, pick a different restaurant.

Digestibles

Be on the lookout for foods prepared by healthful methods such as baking, steaming, broiling, boiling, or grilling. Avoid fried items or those in cream or butter sauce, because those have higher fat content.

To help avoid being swayed by others in your group, order first and stay firm with your order. Remember, the garlic spinach dip may sound great now, but it won't sound so good later when you deal with the aftermath.

If you don't see something IBS-friendly on the menu, ask your server for some help. With the increased awareness of celiac disease and food allergies, most restaurants have no problem making a special effort to ensure your meal is void of onions, provided without a bun, or whatever your heart and intestines desire. Don't hesitate to inquire about the food preparation, ingredients, and menu variations. I always substitute a baked potato for the french fries when possible, and I've never once been yelled at! My husband and I often enjoy splitting an entrée, and at one of our favorite restaurants, the staff has come to ask us if we'll be having the usual "halfners."

Say what you need, and mean what you say. It's really that simple. Remember, when you're dining out at a restaurant, you're paying for a service. Most restaurants want to be sure you leave happy.

Your Best Bets When Dining Out

You may already know your best-tolerated selections when dining out. I know mine. I know pizza isn't a good choice and grilled chicken and a baked potato work well. You may unconsciously know certain foods put you over the edge, and maybe you haven't really thought about it too much. Well, now is the time! Your food diary can help you uncover troublesome foods. While you think about foods that bother you, let's discuss some healthy and tasty selections.

When someone else is doing the cooking, it's hard to know if garlic, onions, and other potentially IBS-irritating ingredients are included. Don't hesitate to ask! The biggest challenge with dining out usually is the portion. Even healthy food choices can be problematic in large quantities. (But now, after reading earlier sections in this chapter, you know how to deal with portions, right?)

Let's look at some different types of restaurants and what some of your best choices are—and what you should avoid.

Your Best Options When Dining Out

Restaurant	Choose	Avoid
Diner	Egg-white omelets, scrambled eggs, pancake, oatmeal	Combo platters with meats, fried eggs, side of home fries

continues

Your Best Options When Dining Out   (continued)

Restaurant	Choose	Avoid
Sandwich shop	Chef salad; grilled chicken salad; pita filled with turkey, ham, roast beef, or grilled chicken	Meatball sub, steak and cheese sub, fried chicken, Italian sub, chicken Parm sub
Asian	Stir-fry with chicken, shrimp, or pork; shrimp with snow peas; beef and broccoli; steamed vegetables; brown rice; sushi	Sweet-and-sour chicken, Peking duck, Kung Pao chicken, fried rice, fried appetizers, tempura, peking ravioli, pu pu platter, crab rangoon
Mexican	Fajitas, soft tacos, arroz con pollo	Chimichangas, bean and cheese dishes, crunchy tacos
Italian	Chicken piccata, chicken marsala, risotto	Fettuccine alfredo, veal or chicken parm, lasagna
Pub/steak house	Filet mignon, grilled fish, grilled chicken, salad with grilled shrimp or chicken	Prime rib, spare ribs, burgers, nachos, fried appetizers

Dining out usually means a fun night out, with a break from cooking and messing up your own kitchen. And you deserve a night off! By choosing wisely and being more aware of what works in your body, you, too, can dine out without consequence!

The Least You Need to Know

◆ Portion control is key to successful dining out while still managing your IBS.

◆ Choose your best-tolerated beverages and limit carbonated beverages, beer with wheat, and soft drinks full of HFCS.

◆ Being more mindful or eating consciously helps you slow down and enjoy your food more.

◆ Preplan what you'd like to eat before you arrive at the restaurant, order first to avoid impulse ordering, and don't hesitate to add special instructions to your order.

Chapter 9

Minimizing Travel Woes

In This Chapter

- ◆ Why travel and IBS don't always mix
- ◆ Essential pack-along foods
- ◆ Tricks to staying hydrated on the road
- ◆ Fitting in fitness

Disrupting your normal schedule and lifestyle can send your IBS body into a tailspin. It's no wonder, as travel generally involves dining out, improper hydration, and minimal exercise—all of which can culminate in the perfect IBS storm. With good advance planning, traveling doesn't need to derail you from your best habits.

Although eating well with IBS on the road may take a bit more thought and pre-trip strategizing, making your due effort will be worth it. In this chapter, you discover how travel disrupts normal digestion and learn what to pack in your IBS-prevention travel kit. So get ready to book your next flight, truly good to go!

Why Travel Makes IBS Worse

A number of factors make your digestive system get a bit out of whack on vacation. If you're traveling by air, bus, train, or car, you're sitting for long periods of time. This idle sitting slows the movement of your intestine, contributing to gas backup and constipation. In other words, a sluggish body leads to a sluggish intestine, which is particularly problematic for the constipation-predominant IBS sufferer.

For you air travelers, air trapped in your intestines can expand during flight. Have you ever brought a small bag of pretzels onboard a plane and noticed that halfway through the flight the bag was blown up like a balloon? (If not, give it a try on your next plane trip!) The same gas expansion can take place in your intestines. Over a long flight, it can be a bit uncomfortable.

Disruptions in your normal eating patterns such as eating Aunt Mary's famous homemade fried chicken and grits can be an unfriendly food environment for you and your IBS. Not being prepared with healthful snacks can lead to your being overhungry and overeating, which culminates in certain malfunction for the IBS belly. And if you're like most folks who travel and don't keep up with your normal exercise routine, this, too, can lead to constipation, bloating, and change in your bowel habits.

Don't be part of the over-under club, those who overeat and underexercise when traveling. Less is not more in this case, and keeping active while traveling is important.

> **Digestibles**
>
> When visiting friends or family, offer to bring a dish with you. Consider preparing a healthful loaf of banana bread or a pasta salad, which you could enjoy with your guests and stick to your IBS-friendly eating plan. Be sure to pack perishables with plenty of ice for food safety.

What to Bring with You

You might have limited space for snacks and IBS supplies, so bring only what you need. If constipation is a problem when you travel, try individually packaged prunes, high-fiber granola bars, high-fiber cereal, and plenty of water for starters. Because of air travel restrictions that don't allow water through security checkpoints, be sure to purchase a large bottle of water after you pass through the metal detectors. You may pay through the roof for it, but hey, you're worth every penny! Estimate about 8 ounces of fluid per hour on a plane because the air is particularly dry up there.

I bring high-fiber granola bars or cereal when I travel. On a recent cruise, I actually brought my cereal with me to the buffet! (High-fiber grains are hard to come by at those buffets.) Learn more about the food options available at your destination prior to your trip so you know what to bring to fill in the gaps. Eating healthy on the road makes for a more pleasant trip because you feel better.

And when it comes to clothes, don't pack or wear your skin-tight jeans when traveling. Clothes that bind around your waist can make your belly feel worse. Instead, opt for loose-fitting, comfy clothes. Loosen the belt a notch, and relax!

Fiber-Filled Snacks

Soluble fiber is generally the best-tolerated fiber for those with IBS, so try to grab granola bars, packets of oatmeal, or cold cereals made with whole oats. You could even bring ground flaxseeds in a zipper-lock bag to use atop your cereal or yogurt.

It may be wise to also keep some psyllium husk or methylcellulose fiber supplements in your toiletry bag in the event that your fiber-rich pack-along foods aren't enough and you need to get things moving.

Some IBS sufferers find that adding FODMAP and fiber-rich foods such as prunes, apples, or pears helps when their body feels like it's backing up. With any increase in fiber foods in your diet, remember that extra fluids help process foods in your body.

 Gut Facts _____

Bringing oat-based cereals on the road with you is easy. Ingredients are listed in order of prevalence in a product, so choose cereals that have whole oats as the first ingredient.

Safe Food Options

You want to feel well while on vacation, so don't let your food choices negatively influence your traveling experience. Try to retain your healthy IBS diet to the best of your ability, and have a little wiggle room for some food indulgences—just try not to go overboard.

While in transit, menu options may be limited, particularly when you're on the road where fast-food joints abound. Try to take a few extra minutes and go off the highway where food options are a bit healthier. If you have one, use your smart phone or PDA to find healthful options nearby, or preplan your stops by searching for restaurants and scanning their menus online prior to hitting the road. This works for me. I'm a picky eater, so I like to have an idea of where I'll be eating while I'm on the road. I usually pack the first meal from home and plan a picnic in the car. For the next meal, I have a preplanned restaurant destination, one that serves healthful food.

Airport food selections can be limited depending on the city and can even vary among terminals. If your plans require a bite at the airport, know what restaurants or vendors are in the terminal. Some options become limited after you pass the security checkpoint, so ask at the information desk before you get through security to find out what food is available and where it is located in the airport.

When you arrive at your destination, food options may get easier, especially if you're visiting at someone's home. If you're at a hotel, you might find a refrigerator in your room (or if not, some hotels will bring one to your room if you request it). If that's not an option, a cooler filled with ice can do for many items you want to keep in your room. When traveling with my family, I always fill our hotel refrigerator with water bottles to ensure we all stay hydrated. Other treats such as yogurt, milk, fruit, granola bars, and cereal are good to have on hand for a light breakfast or mid-afternoon snack.

Probiotics

Remember from Chapter 6 that probiotics are the good bacteria that offer health benefits to your body. Many health professionals recommend you get plenty of probiotics while traveling, especially if disruptions in normal bowel habits are common while you travel.

Gut Facts

Probiotics can be found in yogurt, but also kefir, a dairy drink similar to a fruit smoothie. Kefir is found in health food stores and is available in many fruity flavors.

I enjoy yogurt to get my daily probiotics when I travel and find this helpful for my IBS. Consider trying a daily yogurt with active cultures while you're away from home. Be sure to check the label for "live and active cultures." Those live and active cultures provide the health benefits you want.

Don't Drink the Water

Traveler's diarrhea (TD) is a big problem, particularly for those going to an underdeveloped country. According to the Centers for Disease Control, TD affects 20 to 50 percent of international travelers. A number of conditions can increase your risk of TD, including being a diabetic, taking antacids, having inflammatory bowel disease

(IBS is not inflammatory), or being on medications such as chemotherapy agents that affect your immune system.

The primary source of TD infections is fecally contaminated food or water. Choosing bottled water, not adding ice to your drinks, and sticking with cooked foods are a few ways to lower your risk of TD. Don't assume that you're not at risk just because you're at a resort. Probiotics can help with some forms of diarrhea, but currently there's not enough research to prove it can treat or prevent TD.

Hydrating on the Road

The "don't drink the water in underdeveloped areas" warning in the preceding section notwithstanding, water is your friend in general and especially when traveling. Your brain is 70 percent water and your body around 60 to 65 percent, so water—not soda or other water imposters—is what your body craves. When you're away from home, your faucets, and your fridge, your water consumption can plummet. Water helps move food through the bowel and aids digestion, so not getting enough water can be an issue for the person with IBS.

Drinking more water while traveling may require some preplanning and greater awareness of the role of H_2O in your body. Water is essential for digestion, absorption, and transport of nutrients. Adequate water keeps the mucous membranes, such as the lining of our intestinal tract and skin, moist and supple.

Get more water with these quick and easy tips:

♦ Stop for a decaffeinated iced tea on the go—it's mostly water! Unlike caffeinated tea, which acts like a diuretic causing some water loss, decaffeinated products have a hydrating effect.

♦ Order a fruit salad—fruit contains a lot of water!

♦ Make a point to bring a water bottle on your way out the door.

♦ Bring herbal tea bags with you and just add hot water. On the road, ask for hot water at a restaurant, or run the coffee pot in your hotel room, sans coffee.

♦ Keep a six-pack of water bottles on ice or in the mini bar in your hotel room.

♦ When dining out, ask for refills on the water. Add a lemon or lime wedge for extra flavor!

♦ Always have a water bottle with you on a plane, in a train, or in an automobile.

Don't Forget to Exercise!

Just because you're away from your structured home life doesn't mean you have the right to become a slug. Don't let travel totally disrupt your active lifestyle. You may not keep up with your usual workout schedule, but try to remain active while on the road.

Traveling to get to your new destination can put your activity on hold. Being inactive slows the digestive tract and can contribute to gas buildup and constipation. Exercise has been shown to be helpful in IBS because it helps minimize gas buildup and reduces symptoms, especially in those with abdominal bloating.

Exercise is one of the best lifestyle habits you can do to live a long and healthy life. By now you know the benefits of exercising for IBS, but there are so many other health benefits:

♦ Helps bone health

♦ Lowers blood pressure

♦ Minimizes stress

♦ Helps with sleep

♦ Reduces risk of depression

♦ Decreases risk of heart disease

♦ Lessens risk of cancer

Prior to leaving for your getaway, do a little online research and scope out local gyms, workout facilities, and yoga studios near your destination. Check the hotel website or call the reservation desk to see what types of in-house facilities the hotel offers or if it has arrangements with a local gym. Ask about weekend packages that may include bike rentals.

Here are some more great on-the-road exercise tips:

♦ Take a walking tour of your new destination.

♦ Plan an activity that involves exercise, such as hiking, bike riding, walking, skiing, or swimming.

♦ Skip the cab ride and walk to the restaurant for dinner.

- Pick vacation locations with destinations within walking distance (or just a little beyond if you're feeling adventurous).

- Check out airportgyms.com to see what facilities are available at or near your airport.

- Take a dip in the hotel pool.

- Use the stairs at the hotel.

- Check the television for free exercise videos.

- Bring your significant other along, which may keep you on your regular routine.

 Digestibles

If you have an iPhone, download the Gym Finder app. This free app helps you locate a gym or health club near you, no matter where your destination.

Traveling can disrupt your IBS if you don't manage your diet and exercise plan accordingly. To feel your best, pack snacks and plenty of water. Don't throw all your healthful habits out the window when you travel or you'll likely impact the quality of your time away.

The Least You Need to Know

- Dining out, reduced activity, and inadequate hydration can all impact your IBS when you travel.

- Bring along high-fiber snacks to help manage your fiber intake and offset the risk of travel-related constipation.

- Choose healthful restaurants, and fill your out-of-town refrigerator with IBS-safe foods for snacking or light meals.

- Request extra water at restaurants, and buy some for your hotel room to ensure you get enough much-needed H_2O.

- Keep moving by making prior arrangements for incorporating exercise into your time away from home.

Part 3

Recipes for Eating Well with IBS

You'll never run short on fabulous IBS-friendly dishes with the 160 recipes in Part 3, sure to keep your mouth watering and your IBS in check.

In this part, I give you delicious eggy breakfast favorites, griddle-ready pancakes and breads, hearty and light soups, sandwiches, snacks, and appetizers to please a crowd. You and your family will love the new and different chicken, pork, and beef recipes here, too. And the satisfying seafood selections will keep your heart and brain healthy! There's a little something for everyone's taste buds here, including some great desserts, all designed specifically for you and your IBS body.

Chapter 10

Good Morning Egg Recipes

In This Chapter

- Eggs-cellent protein powerhouses
- Outstanding omelets
- Super stratas and fantastic frittatas
- Delicious quiches and other eggy delights

Starting your day with a nutritious breakfast is an important step in a healthful morning routine. At breakfast, you're literally "breaking the fast" you've encountered during your sleep time. This morning meal doesn't need to be big or overly elaborate. It can be just enough to nourish your body and warm your soul. After a few mornings of a hearty egg break-fast like you'll find in this chapter, you'll come to savor these few quiet moments to indulge your appetite while keeping the symptoms of IBS at bay.

You'll find most of the recipes in this chapter are infused with flavorful vegetables and lean proteins that provide essential vitamins and minerals to keep your body and mind healthy. Let's eat!

Eggs on the Run

Eggs are a complete source of protein, and contain all eight of the food-based essential amino acids your body needs to stay healthy. Each egg has 8 grams of protein, making it a great breakfast choice to jump-start your day.

Eggs also have a great deal of cholesterol, the waxy substance linked with heart disease. The American Heart Association recommends that healthy individuals without elevated LDL cholesterol levels limit cholesterol consumption to 300 milligrams per day. One egg contains approximately 213 milligrams of cholesterol. If consuming eggs in the morning, try to minimize other cholesterol-containing foods that day to keep your cholesterol intake in a healthy range. Other high-cholesterol foods include cheese, butter, whole milk, cream, and beef.

When sitting quietly at the kitchen table at breakfast time just isn't in the cards, grab-and-go dishes are a great option. In this chapter, I've included several nutritious delights you can pack and take with you.

Remember, eggs are perishable and can be a source of food-borne illness, so handle your eggs with care. To be safe, eggs must be cooked until yolks are firm and scrambled eggs are no longer runny. Casseroles such as stratas, frittatas, and quiche dishes should reach an internal temperature of 160°F (use a food thermometer to measure) to ensure thorough cooking.

Quick and Versatile Omelets

You're likely already familiar with omelets. They're like an egg pancake filled with savory ingredients on one side and then gently folded over.

One-egg omelets make a quick-fix breakfast loaded with quality protein. Add a bit of veggies and cheese, and you have quite a nutritious start to your day.

Gut Facts

Legend has it that after a local innkeeper fed Napoleon an omelet, he requested that all the eggs in the village be gathered and made into one large omelet to feed his army.

Rich Stratas and Frittatas

Think of stratas as a flavorful bread-and-egg pudding dish. What's great about stratas is that they can be prepared the night before and popped into the oven the next morning, providing a flavorful and nourishing meal with little morning fuss. Stratas also can easily be made to feed a crowd, and they make a great addition to any brunch or holiday morning meal.

A frittata, on the other hand, is an egg dish made of cheese, eggs, meats, and vegetables. Like stratas, frittatas make a great breakfast and lunchtime menu choice. A slice of frittata is chock-full of protein, vitamins, and minerals. Feel free to mix and match your favorite ingredients or even use last night's leftovers to customize your own strata or frittata!

Digestibles

There's no secret to a perfectly hard-boiled egg. Simply place a few eggs in a single layer in a saucepan, cover with cold water 1 inch higher than the eggs, and set over high heat. When the water boils, remove the pan from the heat, and let the eggs sit in the water for 15 minutes. Immediately run cold water over the eggs and either peel and enjoy right away or refrigerate up to 7 days. Older eggs, about a week to 10 days old, will be easier to peel than fresh eggs.

Cheese and Herb Omelet

This light and cheesy omelet infused with oregano and basil is a delicious way to start your day.

Yield: 1 omelet

Prep time: 5 minutes

Cook time: 3 minutes

Serving size: 1 omelet

Each serving has:

190 calories

1 g carbohydrates

13 g fat

0 g fiber

14 g protein

---

1 tsp. vegetable oil

1 extra-large egg

$\frac{1}{4}$ tsp. Italian seasoning

$\frac{1}{4}$ cup reduced-fat cheddar cheese, grated

1. Add vegetable oil to a small, nonstick skillet, and set over medium heat.

2. In a small bowl, whisk together egg and Italian seasoning. Add egg mixture to the hot skillet, and cook for about 1 minute.

3. Add grated cheese to one side of omelet. Lower heat to medium-low, and cook for about 1 minute.

4. Using a spatula, carefully flip over the side without cheese, making a half circle. Flip omelet completely over, cook for 1 more minute, and serve with whole-grain toast or Brennan's Favorite Home Fries (recipe in Chapter 19).

Variation: To make an extra-hearty omelet, make it a Western Potato Omelet by adding $\frac{1}{2}$ cup cooked hash browns and $\frac{1}{3}$ red pepper to the cheese.

 Gut Facts _____

Cheddar cheese is a great choice for this omelet because it contains no lactose, making this an easy-to-digest morning meal.

Ham and Rosemary Omelet

The savory combination of ham and rosemary pairs deliciously with buttery and nutty cheese in this quick-fix omelet.

1 tsp. vegetable oil

1 extra-large egg

¼ tsp. dried rosemary

¼ cup Swiss cheese, grated

2 slices deli ham, sliced in strips

Yield: 1 omelet
Prep time: 5 minutes
Cook time: 3 minutes
Serving size: 1 omelet
Each serving has:
272 calories
1 g carbohydrates
20 g fat
0 g fiber
24 g protein

1. Add vegetable oil to a small, nonstick skillet, and set over medium heat.

2. In a small bowl, whisk together egg and rosemary. Add egg mixture to the hot skillet, and cook for about 1 minute.

3. Add grated cheese and ham slices to one side of omelet. Lower heat to medium-low, and cook for about 1 minute.

4. Using a spatula, carefully flip over the side without cheese and ham, making a half circle. Flip omelet completely over, cook for 1 more minute, and serve.

Variation: For another tasty combo, make this a **Turkey Bacon and Cheddar Omelet.** Just use 2 slices cooked turkey bacon, cut in 1-inch pieces, and grate ¼ cup cheddar cheese.

Gut Facts

Swiss cheese is a hard cheese, so it has minimal lactose. The holes in Swiss cheese are created by the bacteria that help convert milk into cheese.

Yokeless Wonder Omelet

This light and airy egg-white omelet boasts an Italian flare thanks to the infusion of garlic and basil.

Yield: 1 omelet
Prep time: 5 minutes
Cook time: 3 minutes
Serving size: 1 omelet
Each serving has:
149 calories
5 g carbohydrates
9 g fat
0 g fiber
14 g protein

2 extra-large eggs

¼ tsp. dried basil

¼ tsp. garlic powder

1 tsp. vegetable oil

⅓ cup shredded mozzarella rice cheese

2 medium plum tomatoes, diced (¼ cup)

1. In a small bowl, crack eggs and remove egg yolks, leaving egg whites. (This can be done easily by cracking open egg over a bowl, allowing whites to fall into the bowl, while moving yolk from one eggshell half to the other.) Add basil and garlic powder, and whisk together.

2. Add vegetable oil to a small, nonstick skillet, and set over medium heat.

3. Add egg mixture to the hot skillet, and cook for about 1 minute.

4. Add rice cheese and tomato to one side of omelet. Lower heat to medium-low, and cook for about 1 minute.

5. Using a spatula, carefully flip over the side without cheese and tomatoes, making a half circle. Flip omelet completely over, cook for 1 more minute, and serve.

Digestibles

Traditional mozzarella has some lactose, but shredded rice cheese is a tasty, lactose-free alternative. Shredded mozzarella rice cheese is available at health food stores, but if you can't find it, feel free to substitute grated low-fat cheddar cheese.

The Man Quiche

This flavorful quiche is full of low-fat but savory meats, making it a real man's version of quiche.

1 (9-in.) store-bought piecrust

½ cup cheddar cheese, grated

5 slices turkey bacon, cooked and cut into 1-in. pieces

3 chicken sausages, cooked and cut into bite-size chunks

4 large eggs

1½ cups lactose-free low-fat milk

¼ tsp. onion salt

½ tsp. Italian seasoning

Yield: 1 (9-inch-round) quiche
Prep time: 15 to 20 minutes
Cook time: 40 to 45 minutes
Serving size: ⅙ wedge
Each serving has:
352 calories
19 g carbohydrates
21 g fat
1 g fiber
21 g protein

1. Bake piecrust according to package directions to brown it slightly.

2. Preheat the oven to 375°F.

3. Place cheddar cheese, turkey bacon, and cooked sausage in an even layer in bottom of piecrust.

4. In a medium bowl, whisk together eggs, milk, onion salt, and Italian seasoning. Pour into piecrust, filling just to the top.

5. Bake for 30 minutes or until egg mixture is cooked through. Quiche should be cooked to an internal temperature of 160°F, as measured with a food thermometer.

6. Let sit for 10 minutes to cool down a bit, cut, and serve. If serving with brunch, a garden salad is a great addition.

Gut Facts _____

This hearty quiche is loaded with protein and will appeal to those with large appetites. The lower-fat meats drop the fat content but not the flavor!

Farmer's Muffin Quiche

These muffin quiches are loaded with vegetables and are a great hearty, grab-and-go breakfast.

Yield: 6 quiches
Prep time: 20 to 25 minutes
Cook time: 25 minutes
Serving size: 1 quiche
Each serving has:
110 calories
3 g carbohydrates
7 g fat
1 g fiber
8 g protein

Gut Facts

These quiches are handy to keep in the refrigerator for rushed morning meals. They make a great after-school snack or a part of a healthy lunch, too!

3 large eggs

¾ cup reduced-lactose low-fat milk

½ tsp. garlic powder

1 TB. vegetable oil

1 small tomato, chopped and seeded

1 cup broccoli, florets and stems, finely chopped

1 cup button mushrooms, finely chopped

½ cup reduced-fat cheddar cheese, grated

2 TB. chopped fresh basil

1. Preheat the oven to 350°F. Spray 6 muffin tins with nonstick cooking spray.

2. In a medium bowl, whisk together eggs, milk, and garlic powder. Set aside.

3. Add vegetable oil to a medium, nonstick skillet, and set over medium heat. Add tomato, broccoli, and mushrooms, and sauté for about 5 minutes or until vegetables are fork-tender. Carefully drain all extra liquid from vegetables.

4. Spread egg mixture evenly among muffin cups, filling each about ½ full. Top each muffin cup with 1 spoonful vegetable mixture, add 1 spoonful cheese, and garnish with pinch of basil. Bake for 20 minutes or until eggs are set.

5. Run a butter knife around edge of each quiche, and let sit in the tin for 2 or 3 minutes before serving.

Ham and Cheese Strata

Nutty cheese mingles with savory meat, making this strata perfectly flavorful.

½ (6- to 8-in.) French baguette

½ cup Swiss cheese, grated

1 cup cubed ham chunks

1 cup reduced-lactose low-fat milk

4 large eggs

1 tsp. dry mustard

½ tsp. onion salt

1 tsp. dried basil

¼ tsp. freshly ground black pepper

1 TB. chopped fresh parsley

Yield: 1 (8×8-inch) strata
Prep time: 10 minutes plus overnight refrigeration time
Cook time: 35 minutes
Serving size: ¼-strata square
Each serving has:
257 calories
17.5 g carbohydrates
12 g fat
<1 g fiber
20 g protein

1. Spray an 8×8-inch-square pan with nonstick cooking spray.

2. Cut French baguette into 1-inch cubes, and arrange in a single layer in the prepared pan. Top with Swiss cheese and ham chunks.

3. In a medium bowl, whisk together milk, eggs, dry mustard, onion salt, basil, and pepper. Pour egg mixture over bread in pan. Cover with plastic wrap, and refrigerate overnight.

4. The next day, preheat the oven to 350°F. Top strata with chopped parsley, and bake, uncovered, for 30 minutes or until puffed and slightly browned on edges. Center should be cooked through. Let sit for 10 minutes prior to slicing and serving.

 Digestibles

This recipe works well with leftover ham, but if you don't have any, ask at your deli for a 1-inch chunk of ham. You can then easily cut it into chunks for this strata.

Spinach and Parmesan Strata

Earthy spinach complements tangy Parmesan cheese in this rich and filling strata.

Yield: 1 (8×8-inch) strata
Prep time: 10 minutes plus overnight refrigeration time
Cook time: 35 minutes
Serving size: ¼ strata square
Each serving has:
255 calories
20 g carbohydrates
12 g fat
3 g fiber
19 g protein

½ (6- to 8-in.) French baguette

½ cup Parmesan cheese, grated

1¼ cups frozen chopped spinach, cooked and drained

1 cup reduced-lactose low-fat milk

4 large eggs

¼ tsp. ground nutmeg

½ tsp. garlic salt

¼ tsp. freshly ground black pepper

1. Spray an 8×8-inch-square pan with nonstick cooking spray.

2. Cut French baguette into 1-inch cubes, and arrange in a single layer in the prepared pan. Top with Parmesan cheese and cooked spinach.

3. In a medium bowl, whisk together milk, eggs, nutmeg, garlic salt, and pepper. Pour egg mixture over bread in pan. Cover with plastic wrap, and refrigerate overnight.

4. The next day, preheat the oven to 350°F. Bake strata, uncovered, for 30 minutes or until puffed and slightly browned on edges. Center should be cooked through. Let sit for 10 minutes prior to slicing and serving.

Gut Facts

Spinach is chock-full of good nutrition, including calcium, vitamins A and C, iron, potassium, and even magnesium. Popeye knew what he was doing—spinach is a super food!

Broccoli and Cheddar Strata

This flavorful strata is a hearty breakfast dish and a great way to slip in another serving of broccoli into your diet.

$\frac{1}{2}$ (6- to 8-in.) French baguette

$\frac{1}{2}$ cup reduced-fat cheddar cheese, grated

2 cups frozen chopped broccoli, cooked and drained

1 cup reduced-lactose low-fat milk

4 large eggs

1 tsp. dry mustard

$\frac{1}{2}$ tsp. garlic salt

$\frac{1}{4}$ tsp. freshly ground black pepper

1 TB. chopped fresh parsley

Yield: 1 (8×8-inch) strata
Prep time: 10 minutes plus overnight refrigeration time
Cook time: 35 minutes
Serving size: $\frac{1}{4}$ strata square
Each serving has:
229 calories
19 g carbohydrates
10 g fat
1 g fiber
17 g protein

1. Spray an 8×8-inch-square pan with nonstick cooking spray.

2. Cut French baguette into 1-inch cubes, and arrange in a single layer in the prepared pan. Top with cheddar cheese and broccoli.

3. In a medium bowl, whisk together milk, eggs, dry mustard, garlic salt, pepper, and parsley. Pour egg mixture over bread in pan. Cover with plastic wrap, and refrigerate overnight.

4. The next day, preheat the oven to 350°F. Bake strata, uncovered, for 30 minutes or until puffed and slightly browned on edges. Center should be cooked through. Let sit for 10 minutes prior to slicing and serving.

Tummy Trouble

Broccoli is from the cruciferous vegetable family well known for its anti-cancer properties. Too much broccoli can cause gas, so be sure to stick to the recommended portion size serving.

Tomato and Cheese Frittata

There's nothing like the tangy and creamy combination of cheese and tomatoes, making this frittata a delicious way to start your day.

Yield: 6 servings
Prep time: 5 minutes
Cook time: 26 minutes
Serving size: $\frac{1}{6}$ frittata wedge
Each serving has:
169 calories
4 g carbohydrates
11 g fat
1 g fiber
13 g protein

$1\frac{1}{2}$ **cups grape tomatoes, cut in half**

1 tsp. vegetable oil

1 tsp. onion powder

8 large eggs

1 cup cheddar cheese

1 TB. chopped fresh parsley

1. Preheat the oven to 350°F.

2. In 10-inch ovenproof skillet over medium heat, sauté tomatoes with vegetable oil and onion powder for about 2 minutes or until tomatoes are soft. Drain extra liquid from the skillet.

3. In a medium bowl, whisk eggs until well blended. Pour eggs into the skillet, over vegetables (no need to stir), and sprinkle with cheddar cheese and parsley. Cook for 6 minutes.

4. Place skillet in the oven, and bake for 20 minutes. Let cool for 5 minutes, cut into 6 wedges, and serve.

Gut Facts

Tomatoes are rich in lycopene, a phytochemical (plant chemical) found in red-colored fruits and vegetables, that's linked with lowering risk of cancer, especially prostate, lung, and stomach cancers.

Grated Zucchini and Roasted Red Bell Pepper Frittata

Here, the mild-flavored veggies and garlic complement the egg in a nice, understated way.

1 medium zucchini, diced small

1 large roasted red bell pepper, cut into 1-in. strips

1 TB. vegetable oil

½ tsp. garlic powder

8 large eggs

1 cup reduced-fat cheddar cheese, grated

1 TB. chopped fresh parsley

Yield: 6 wedge slices
Prep time: 5 minutes
Cook time: 30 minutes
Serving size: ⅙ frittata wedge
Each serving has:
187 calories
4 g carbohydrates
12 g fat
1 g fiber
14 g protein

1. Preheat the oven to 350°F.

2. In 10-inch ovenproof skillet over medium heat, sauté zucchini and roasted red bell pepper with vegetable oil and garlic powder for about 6 minutes, stirring often, or until vegetables are soft. Drain any excess liquid from the skillet.

3. In medium bowl, whisk eggs until well blended. Pour into the skillet, and sprinkle cheddar cheese and parsley over top. Cook for about 4 minutes.

4. Place skillet in the oven, and bake for 20 minutes. Let cool for about 5 minutes, cut into 6 wedges, and serve.

Digestibles

You can find roasted red bell peppers in the international or Italian section of most grocery stores.

Breakfast Sandwich to Go

This hearty quick-fix breakfast sandwich incorporates tangy tomato with flavorful ham and sharp cheddar cheese.

Yield: 1 sandwich
Prep time: 5 minutes
Cook time: 2 minutes
Serving size: 1 sandwich
Each serving has:
381 calories
32 g carbohydrates
17 g fat
2 g fiber
25 g protein

1 extra-large egg

1 slice sharp cheddar cheese

1 slice deli ham

1 whole-wheat English muffin

1 slice tomato

1. In small, microwave-safe bowl, beat egg with a fork. Microwave on high for 30 seconds, remove carefully, and stir.

2. Place cheese and ham slices over egg, and return to the microwave. Cook for another 30 seconds, or until egg is no longer runny.

3. Meanwhile, toast English muffin.

4. Remove egg dish from the microwave and, using a spoon, carefully scoop out egg, ham, and cheese and place on one half of toasted English muffin.

5. Add tomato slice, and top with other half of English muffin, and serve.

 Digestibles _____

Microwaves vary, so adjust the cooking time as necessary so your egg is thoroughly cooked but not overcooked.

Scrambled Olé Burrito

After one bite, you'll swear you were in a small Mexican village enjoying this egg dish with a kick of chili powder!

1 large egg

¼ tsp. chili powder (optional; eliminate if it bothers you)

1 (10-in.) brown rice tortilla

¼ cup reduced-fat cheddar cheese, grated

1 TB. salsa

Yield: 1 burrito
Prep time: 2 minutes
Cook time: 2 or 3 minutes
Serving size: 1 burrito
Each serving has:
294 calories
26 g carbohydrates
13 g fat
3 g fiber
17 g protein

1. In a small bowl, whisk together egg and chili powder (if using).

2. Heat a small, nonstick skillet over medium heat. Add egg mixture, and cook for 1 or 2 minutes, scrambling with a fork, until egg is cooked through and no longer runny.

3. Place brown rice tortilla on a microwave-safe plate, top with cheese and salsa, and microwave on high for 10 to 15 seconds. Remove from the microwave.

4. Place scrambled egg on top of cheese mixture. Fold tortilla in half, carefully fold in sides just about 2 inches toward center of tortilla, and, while holding the folded ends, roll tortilla over. Voilà!

 Digestibles _____

If the onions in salsa are problematic for you, try a spoonful of diced tomatoes with 1 tablespoon chopped fresh cilantro and a splash of fresh lemon juice from ½ lemon.

Your Daily Breads (and Grains)

In This Chapter

- ◆ Perfect pancakes
- ◆ Delicious breakfast breads
- ◆ Bowl- and belly-filling oatmeal
- ◆ Simple homemade nutty granola

There's nothing quite like some yummy pancakes or sweet breakfast breads or muffins to quell a morning sweet tooth. This chapter's quick-fix breads, pancakes, and muffin recipes are often wheat free, which will please not only your sweet tooth but also your belly. Other recipes have modified amounts of wheat to keep often-troublesome fructans at a minimum.

These breakfast delights also contain lots of oats, making them very belly-friendly. If you're short on time, try the Creamy Slow Cooker Oatmeal that cooks while you sleep. And for a nutritious breakfast on the go, nutty homemade granola makes a great addition to any morning routine. Mix it with your favorite yogurt and fruits, and you're ready to hit the road!

Banana Pancakes

These quick-fix treats are like banana bread in a pancake form. *(Adapted and reprinted with permission from IBSFree.net by Patsy Catsos, R.D.)*

Yield: 12 small pancakes
Prep time: 5 minutes
Cook time: 4 minutes per batch
Serving size: 2 pancakes
Each serving has:
137 calories
17 g carbohydrates
4 g fat
2 g fiber
9 g protein

1 cup regular or gluten-free *old-fashioned oats*

1 cup lactose-free low-fat cottage cheese

3 large eggs

1 large ripe banana, peeled

1 tsp. ground cinnamon

1. In a blender, add old-fashioned oats, cottage cheese, eggs, banana, and cinnamon. Blend for about 90 seconds or until smooth. (Be sure cottage cheese especially is smooth.)

2. Lightly spray a medium, nonstick skillet with nonstick cooking spray and set over medium heat.

3. When skillet is hot, add pancake batter by the ¼ cup. Cook for about 2 minutes or until edges are dry and tops are starting to set. Flip over pancakes using a spatula. Cook for about 2 more minutes or until pancake is puffed up in the middle. Place cooked pancakes on a serving platter, and cover with aluminum foil to keep warm while you cook remaining pancakes.

4. Serve with real maple syrup.

 Wellness Words

> **Old-fashioned oats** or rolled oats are used in this and the majority of the recipes in this book. These whole oats have been rolled and flaked, and they add a bit of a nutty texture. Instant oats are cut in smaller bits, making them cook quicker and add less texture to recipes, but in a pinch, they can be substituted.

Pumpkin Spice Pancakes

With these pancakes reminiscent of pumpkin pie, you can enjoy the taste of fall all year round.

1 cup oat flour	**½ tsp. pumpkin pie spice**
½ cup all-purpose flour	**½ cup canned pumpkin**
1 TB. sugar	**2 eggs**
2½ tsp. baking powder	**¾ cup reduced-lactose low-fat milk**

1. In a medium bowl, lightly combine oat flour, all-purpose flour, sugar, baking powder, and pumpkin pie spice.

2. In a small bowl, mix pumpkin, eggs, and milk. Add pumpkin mixture to flour mixture, and blend with spoon by hand until free of lumps.

3. Lightly spray a medium, nonstick skillet with nonstick cooking spray and set over medium heat.

4. When skillet is hot, add pancake batter by the ¼ cup. Cook for about 2 minutes or until edges are dry and tops are starting to set. Flip over pancakes using a spatula. Cook for about 2 more minutes or until pancake is puffed up in the middle. Place cooked pancakes on a serving platter, and cover with aluminum foil to keep warm while you cook remaining pancakes.

5. Serve with a drizzle of warm maple syrup with 1 tablespoon chopped pecans.

Yield: 12 medium pancakes

Prep time: 10 minutes

Cook time: 4 minutes per batch

Serving size: 2 pancakes

Each serving has:

148 calories

21 g carbohydrates

3.5 g fat

2 g fiber

7 g protein

 Gut Facts

Pumpkin is a great source of fiber and vitamin A. Vitamin A keeps your immune system strong and also helps you see well at night.

Russell T. Blueberry Pancakes

My husband, Russ, likes just about any food that has blueberries in it, and these very-blueberry pancakes are his favorite.

Yield: 8 small pancakes
Prep time: 10 minutes
Cook time: 4 minutes per batch
Serving size: 2 small pancakes
Each serving has:
160 calories
29 g carbohydrates
2 g fat
2 g fiber
3 g protein

½ cup unbleached white flour
½ cup oat flour
1½ TB. sugar
2 tsp. baking powder
½ tsp. baking soda

¼ tsp. salt
½ cup vanilla rice milk
1 tsp. vegetable oil
1 tsp. vanilla extract
¾ cup fresh blueberries

1. In a medium mixing bowl, combine white flour, oat flour, sugar, baking powder, baking soda, and salt.

2. Add vanilla rice milk, vegetable oil, and vanilla extract, and stir until well blended and free of lumps.

3. Gently add blueberries, and mix lightly until evenly distributed.

4. Spray a large skillet with nonstick cooking spray, and set over medium heat.

5. When skillet is hot, add pancake batter by the ¼ cup. Cook for about 2 minutes or until edges are dry and tops are starting to set. Flip over pancakes using a spatula. Cook for about 2 more minutes or until pancake is puffed up in the middle. Place cooked pancakes on a serving platter, and cover with aluminum foil to keep warm while you cook remaining pancakes.

6. Serve as desired. We like a bit of butter and confectioners' sugar sprinkled on top.

Digestibles

Rice milk has no lactose, so it's easier on your belly. The protein content tends to be far lower than cow's milk, so be sure to get other protein in your diet when substituting with rice milk.

Vanilla-Cinnamon French Toast

A pure and natural blend of vanilla combines with the subtle sweetness of cinnamon to make this French toast tops on the "comfort food" list.

1 tsp. butter or trans-fat-free margarine

2 tsp. vegetable oil

1 large egg

½ cup reduced-lactose low-fat milk

1 tsp. vanilla extract

Dash ground cinnamon

4 slices whole-grain bread

Yield: 4 slices
Prep time: 5 minutes
Cook time: 6 minutes
Serving size: 2 slices
Each serving has:
260 calories
32 g carbohydrates
10 g fat
4 g fiber
11 g protein

1. In a large skillet over medium heat, add margarine and vegetable oil.

2. In a medium bowl, whisk together egg, milk, vanilla extract, and cinnamon.

3. Dip bread into egg mixture, turning over to coat both sides. Place bread in the skillet. Repeat with remaining slices.

4. Cook for 2 or 3 minutes or until lightly browned, flip over, and cook the other side for 2 or 3 more minutes.

5. Serve with maple syrup and sliced strawberries, or sprinkle with confectioners' sugar.

Digestibles

Feel free to substitute your favorite bread in this dish. It will add a bit of variety and flavor depending on the bread you use.

Squash Bread

Similar to its cousin pumpkin bread, this sweet fall treat is fabulous with a hint of cinnamon.

Yield: 12 *slices*
Prep time: 10 minutes
Cook time: 55 minutes
Serving size: 1 slice
Each serving has:
242 calories
33 g carbohydrates
10 g fat
2 g fiber
4 g protein

 Gut Facts

Canned squash is often found in the baking aisle next to the canned pumpkin.

1 (15-oz.) can squash	½ cup oat flour
1 cup sugar	1 tsp. baking soda
½ cup vegetable oil	¼ tsp. salt
2 large eggs	¾ tsp. ground cinnamon
1¼ cups unbleached all-purpose flour	2 TB. unsalted pumpkin seeds

1. Preheat the oven to 350°F. Spray a 9×5×3 loaf pan with nonstick cooking spray.

2. In a medium bowl, combine squash, sugar, vegetable oil, and eggs with a fork until smooth and well blended.

3. Add all-purpose flour, oat flour, baking soda, salt, and cinnamon, and mix well.

4. Pour batter into the prepared pan, top evenly with pumpkin seeds, and bake for 55 minutes or until a toothpick inserted in the center comes out clean. For a softer crust, cover top of loaf with aluminum foil after 35 minutes of cook time.

Orange Chocolate-Chip Muffins

The orange and chocolate fusion in these muffins is a wonderful blend.

1 cup white rice flour	**2 TB. vegetable oil**
2 TB. cornstarch	**1 large egg**
½ tsp. baking soda	**¼ cup orange juice**
½ tsp. ground cinnamon	**½ cup mini semi-sweet chocolate chips**
¼ cup sugar	

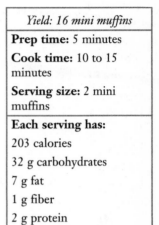

Yield: 16 mini muffins
Prep time: 5 minutes
Cook time: 10 to 15 minutes
Serving size: 2 mini muffins
Each serving has:
203 calories
32 g carbohydrates
7 g fat
1 g fiber
2 g protein

1. Preheat the oven to 350°F. Fill a mini muffin tin with 16 mini muffin liners.

2. In a medium bowl, combine rice flour, cornstarch, baking soda, cinnamon, and sugar. Add vegetable oil, egg, and orange juice, and blend well. Gently mix in chocolate chips.

3. Pour batter into mini muffin cups, filling each about ¾ full.

4. Bake for 10 to 15 minutes or until a toothpick inserted in the center comes out clean. Serve warm.

Gut Facts

For some IBS sufferers, rice flour can be easier on the belly than wheat flour because it doesn't contain troublesome fructans. Plus, it provides a light texture to wheat-free baked goods.

Creamy Slow Cooker Oatmeal

I love waking up to this nutty oatmeal on cold winter mornings.

Yield: 4 cups
Prep time: 3 minutes
Cook time: 8 hours or overnight
Serving size: 1 cup
Each serving has:
150 calories
27 g carbohydrates
2.5 g fat
4 g fiber
6 g protein

1 cup *steel-cut oats*   1 tsp. ground cinnamon

4¾ cups water

1. The night before, pour steel-cut oats, water, and cinnamon into a slow cooker, and give a big stir. Cover, and set heat to low.

2. The next morning, whisk oatmeal before serving.

Variation: This oatmeal is delicious as is, but you might also like **Sweet 'n' Fruity Slow Cooker Oatmeal.** Simply add 2 tablespoons almonds, ¼ cup fresh blueberries,, a drizzle of maple syrup, or 1 teaspoon brown sugar—or all of the above—to the hot, cooked oatmeal and enjoy!

Wellness Words _____

Steel-cut oats are a very hearty form of oatmeal high in fiber and protein. Steel-cut oats are whole-grain oats taken from the inner part of the oat kernel. Cooking the oats in a slow cooker overnight allows for a quick breakfast without the morning fuss.

Wheat-Free Vanilla-Almond Granola

The sweet and nutty almond flavor and aroma of this homemade granola is a terrific way to start your day.

3 cups old-fashioned oats

½ cup oat bran

1 cup sliced almonds, coarsely chopped

¼ cup unsalted raw or roasted sunflower seeds

1 tsp. ground cinnamon

1 tsp. vanilla extract

¼ tsp. coconut or almond extract (your choice)

½ cup maple syrup

¼ cup vegetable oil

Yield: 4 cups
Prep time: 10 minutes
Cook time: 40 minutes
Serving size: ¼ cup
Each serving has:
167 calories
20 g carbohydrates
14 g fat
3 g fiber
4 g protein

1. Preheat the oven to 300°F. Spray an 11×15-inch jelly-roll pan or a cookie sheet with edges with nonstick cooking spray.

2. In a large bowl, combine oats, oat bran, almonds, sunflower seeds, and cinnamon.

3. In a small bowl, combine vanilla extract, coconut extract, maple syrup, and vegetable oil. Drizzle over oat mixture, and stir until combined.

4. Spread granola in an even layer on the prepared jelly-roll pan, and place in the oven. Cook for 40 minutes, stirring every 10 minutes to ensure even cooking, until granola is toasted light brown. Store in airtight container for 7 to 10 days.

Digestibles

Enjoy this whole-grain granola in a yogurt parfait (recipes in Chapter 12), with reduced-lactose milk, or take with you as a good grab-and-go snack.

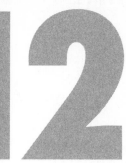

Chapter 12

Breakfast Smoothies and Parfaits

In This Chapter

- ◆ Berry delicious smoothies
- ◆ Frozen citrus-y concoctions
- ◆ Hearty fruit and yogurt parfaits

Smoothies work well for the IBS body and are a great way to add fruit to your diet. Most Americans fall short on fruit consumption, and we all know how much your body craves fruits and vegetables for optimal health. Fruity, creamy smoothies are a fine way to start your day. So power up your blender and let's get the (smoothie) party started!

But let's not overlook parfaits. Parfaits make a tasty and nutritious breakfast meal, thanks to the protein from the yogurt and a hearty dose of fiber from the granola. Nuts lower risk of high blood pressure and heart disease, so fruit parfaits made with nut-filled whole-grain granola keep your ticker happy, too. Enjoy these crunchy delights at the breakfast table or pack one to go on your more rushed mornings.

Berry Good Smoothie

The mixed berries in this smoothie burst with fruity goodness and will make your mouth happy.

Yield: 3 cups
Prep time: 5 minutes
Serving size: 1 cup
Each serving has:
102 calories
18 g carbohydrates
0 g fat
3 g fiber
7 g protein

2 cups frozen mixed berries

¼ cup water

1 cup vanilla nonfat Greek yogurt

1. In a blender, combine mixed berries, water, and yogurt.

2. Blend on high speed for about 15 seconds. Stop the blender, stir mixture, and blend again until smoothie is creamy and smooth. Serve immediately.

Gut Facts

Greek yogurt has a creamier consistency than other yogurts. The protein content is also considerably higher, making this smoothie really stick to your ribs. Greek yogurt is strained longer than conventional yogurt, which gives it a creamier texture.

Sassy Strawberry Smoothie

There's nothing more delightful than the sweet taste of summer fruits with a hint of vanilla.

2 cups frozen whole strawberries

¾ cup water

1 cup vanilla nonfat Greek yogurt

Yield: *3 cups*
Prep time: 5 minutes
Serving size: 1 cup
Each serving has:
87 calories
14 g carbohydrates
0 g fat
2 g fiber
7 g protein

1. In a blender, combine strawberries, water, and yogurt.

2. Blend on high speed for about 15 seconds. Stop the blender, stir mixture, and blend again until smoothie is creamy and smooth. Serve immediately.

 Gut Facts _____

Strawberries are a great source of vitamin C, which helps the body absorb iron from foods, heals the skin, and likely lowers the risk of cancer and heart disease.

Banana Smoothie

This creamy smoothie tastes like a fruity vanilla milkshake—with banana, too, of course!

Yield: 3 cups
Prep time: 5 minutes
Serving size: 1 cup
Each serving has:
120 calories
24 g carbohydrates
0 g fat
2 g fiber
6 g protein

2 frozen extra-ripe medium bananas

¼ cup water

1 cup vanilla nonfat Greek yogurt

1. In a blender, combine bananas, water, and yogurt.

2. Blend on high speed for about 15 seconds. Stop the blender, stir mixture, and blend again until smoothie is creamy and smooth. Serve immediately.

Digestibles

Let bananas ripen on the kitchen countertop until small brown dots appear. Then you can peel the bananas and place them in the freezer for later use in smoothies. Ripe bananas are easier to digest and better tolerated in IBS. Bananas are a great source of potassium.

Frozen Blueberry-Lemon Smoothie

Sweet and sour unite in this tart smoothie to make your mouth water just thinking about it.

¾ cup lemon nonfat yogurt   Water

1½ cups frozen blueberries

1. In a blender, combine yogurt and blueberries.

2. Blend on high speed for about 15 seconds. Stop the blender, stir mixture, add a bit of water to thin if necessary, and blend again until smoothie is creamy and smooth. Serve immediately.

Gut Facts

Thanks to their anti-inflammatory properties, blueberries are a good choice for conditions linked with inflammation such as heart disease and arthritis.

Yield: 2 cups
Prep time: 5 minutes
Serving size: 1 cup
Each serving has:
129 calories
29 g carbohydrates
1 g fat
4 g fiber
4 g protein

Orange Creamsicle Delight

This smoothie is just like the creamsicles the ice-cream man delivers in the summertime—but a whole lot better for you!

½ cup orange juice	**1 cup ice**
1 cup vanilla nonfat Greek yogurt	

Yield: 2 cups
Prep time: 5 minutes
Serving size: 1 cup
Each serving has:
100 calories
15 g carbohydrates
0 g fat
0 g fiber
10 g protein

1. In a blender, combine orange juice, yogurt, and ice.

2. Blend on high speed for about 15 seconds. Stop the blender, stir mixture, and blend again until smoothie is creamy and smooth. Serve immediately.

Gut Facts

Orange juice is a great source of vitamin C, potassium, and folate. Use OJ fortified with calcium and vitamin D for an extra boost of these bone-friendly nutrients.

Kool Kiwifruit Kooler

This smoothie is a sweet and tangy delight, thanks to the combination of kiwifruit and blueberry yogurt.

2 medium kiwifruit, peeled   **2 cups ice**

1 cup blueberry nonfat Greek yogurt

1. In a blender, combine kiwifruit, yogurt, and ice.

2. Blend on high speed for about 15 seconds. Stop the blender, stir mixture, and blend again until smoothie is creamy and smooth. Serve immediately.

Gut Facts

Did you know kiwifruits are also known as Chinese gooseberries? They're also a top source of vitamin C.

Yield: 2 cups
Prep time: 5 minutes
Serving size: 1 cup
Each serving has:
136 calories
23 g carbohydrates
0 g fat
2 g fiber
11 g protein

Citrus Surprise

This refreshing drink is full of citrus-y tang with a clean lemon finish.

Yield: 3 cups
Prep time: 5 minutes
Serving size: 1 cup
Each serving has:
63 calories
13 g carbohydrates
0 g fat
0 g fiber
3 g protein

$\frac{1}{2}$ **cup orange juice**   **2 cups ice**

$\frac{3}{4}$ **cup lemon nonfat yogurt**

1. In a blender, combine orange juice, yogurt, and ice.

2. Blend on high speed for about 15 seconds. Stop the blender, stir mixture, and blend again until smoothie is creamy and smooth. Serve immediately.

Gut Facts

According to the World Health Organization, worldwide inadequate fruit and vegetable intake is estimated to cause about 19 percent of gastrointestinal cancer, about 31 percent of ischemic heart disease, and 11 percent of stroke. So drink up!

Berry-Deelish Granola-Strawberry Parfait

Sun-ripened sweetness meets vanilla cream with a nice crunch finish in this wholesome breakfast parfait.

2 cups vanilla nonfat Greek yogurt

1 cup strawberries, hulled and sliced

1 cup blueberries

½ cup granola

Yield: 2 parfaits	
Prep time: 5 minutes	
Serving size: 1 parfait	
Each serving has:	
377 calories	
51 g carbohydrates	
14.5 g fat	
7 g fiber	
25 g protein	

1. Into 2 (16-ounce) serving glasses, spoon ½ cup yogurt, ¼ cup strawberries, and ¼ cup blueberries. Repeat with remaining yogurt and berries.

2. Top each with ¼ cup granola, and serve.

 Digestibles _____

You could use store-bought granola in these parfaits, but why not try my Wheat-Free Vanilla-Almond Granola (recipe in Chapter 11)? And for the berries, if you can't find fresh, you can use frozen. Just defrost them in the refrigerator the night before using.

Almond-Vanilla-Blueberry Parfait

Here, whole-grain goodness teams up with a bit of sweet and nutty flavor.

Yield: 2 parfaits
Prep time: 5 minutes
Serving size: 1 parfait
Each serving has:
458 calories
49 g carbohydrates
23 g fat
7 g fiber
28 g protein

2 cups vanilla nonfat Greek yogurt

¼ cup sliced almonds

1 cup frozen blueberries

½ cup Wheat-Free Vanilla-Almond Granola (recipe in Chapter 11)

1. In a blender, combine yogurt, almonds, and blueberries.

2. Blend on high speed for about 15 seconds. Stop the blender, stir mixture, and blend again until mixture is creamy and smooth.

3. Divide yogurt mixture between 2 glass dishes. Top each with ¼ cup Wheat-Free Vanilla-Almond Granola, and serve.

Gut Facts

Thanks to the almonds, this parfait has lots of monounsaturated fat—the most heart-friendly fat. A diet rich in nuts has been linked with lowering blood fats and risk of heart disease. Enjoy this nutty parfait while keeping your heart happy!

Chapter 13

Super Snacks and Starters

In This Chapter

- Fruit- and veggie-rich dips
- Scrumptious salsas
- Protein-packed appetizers
- Snazzy snacks everyone will love

Grazing—snacking on healthful dips, snacks, and mini meals throughout the day—is a great way to meet your nutritional needs while keeping your IBS symptoms at bay. Many of the recipes are chock-full of fruits and vegetables to keep your belly healthy.

You can mix and match the fabulous snacks in this chapter during the week to jazz up your regular snacking routine, or you can prepare them for your next gathering and really wow your guests! The recipes may take you outside of your typical recipe box, but have no fear. They'll become your new favorites.

Ready? It's time to snack!

A Few Notes on Noshing

The dips, spreads, salsas, and appetizers in this chapter serve up a lot of flavorful goodness. Many can be made ahead and simply reheated when you want a bite-size morsel of healthy goodness through the week. They make great in-between mealtime fillers, too.

Spreads and dips are terrific served with crackers, tortilla chips, or fresh-cut veggies. They also make a great addition to your favorite sandwich or wrap.

Colorful, tangy, low-calorie salsas are just what you need to make grilled fish or chicken go from mundane to spectacular. Enjoy the fruit salsas over angel food cake for a quick and fancy dessert. Salsas can be prepared in advance and stored safely in your fridge for up to three or four days.

My favorite might be bite-size appetizers. They're so easy to deal with when entertaining! And they're versatile enough, they make a great everyday snack or can knock the socks off your dinner guests. Time to start planning your next party!

Gut Facts

Salsas are rich in vibrant fruits and vegetables. What a tasty way to get your body's necessary vitamins and minerals!

Guacamole

This fresh lemony and garlic dip makes a quick and colorful appetizer. *(Reprinted with permission from IBSFree.net by Patsy Catsos, R.D.)*

2 ripe avocados

Juice of 1 large lemon

1 clove garlic, sliced large

¼ tsp. salt

¼ tsp. freshly ground black pepper

¼ cup chopped fresh cilantro

Yield: 2 cups, 8 servings
Prep time: 25 minutes
Serving size: ¼ cup
Each serving has:
86 calories
5 g carbohydrates
7.5 g fat
3 g fiber
1 g protein

1. Peel avocados, and cut in half. Remove and discard seed. Scoop out flesh, and place it in small mixing bowl.

2. Drizzle lemon juice over top of avocado, and add garlic slices, salt, and pepper, and gently stir.

3. Cover the bowl with plastic wrap and refrigerate for 15 minutes.

4. Remove garlic slices, mash mixture, top with cilantro, and serve with tortilla chips.

 Tummy Trouble

Garlic is a member of the fructan family, so it might be irritating to your IBS. In lieu of a fresh garlic clove, feel free to substitute ⅛ teaspoon garlic powder, which you can leave in the finished product.

Cheesy Dill Dip

This cheese-y, garlic-y, dill-y dip won't last very long after you serve it to your guests!

Yield: 1 cup, 4 servings
Prep time: 5 minutes
Serving size: ¼ cup
Each serving has:
40 calories
1.5 g carbohydrates
0.5 g fat
0 g fiber
7 g protein

1 cup reduced-lactose low-fat cottage cheese

1½ tsp. dried dill

½ tsp. garlic salt

2 TB. chopped fresh parsley

1. In a blender, combine cottage cheese, dill, garlic salt, and parsley.

2. Blend on medium speed for 3 to 5 minutes or until creamy.

3. Serve with baby carrots, sliced red peppers, or rice crackers.

Gut Facts

You can find reduced-lactose cottage cheese in most larger grocery stores these days. Look in the dairy case.

Lemon-Eggplant Dip

This savory dip is full of creamy, lemon-y goodness!

1 large eggplant

2 tsp. plus 1 TB. olive oil

2 cloves garlic, peeled and cut in half

3 TB. freshly squeezed lemon juice (about 1 lemon)

3 TB. *tahini*

½ tsp. garlic salt

1 TB. chopped fresh parsley

Yield: 2 cups, 8 servings
Prep time: 10 minutes
Cook time: 50 to 60 minutes
Serving size: ¼ cup
Each serving has:
80 calories
6 g carbohydrates
7 g fat
1 g fiber
1 g protein

1. Preheat the oven to 350°F.

2. Cut stem off eggplant, and cut eggplant in half. Drizzle flesh with 2 teaspoons olive oil and top with garlic. Wrap eggplant, cut sides facing each other, with aluminum foil, and place on a cookie sheet. Roast for 50 to 60 minutes or until fork-tender.

3. Remove from the oven and let cool enough to handle.

4. Scoop out eggplant flesh into a medium bowl, discarding garlic and eggplant skin. Mash flesh with a fork until smooth. (For extra-smooth consistency, add to a blender or food processor, fitted with metal blade attachment, and blend for 1 minute.)

5. Add lemon juice, tahini, and garlic salt, and mix well. Place in the serving dish.

6. Drizzle remaining 1 tablespoon olive oil over top, garnish with parsley, and serve.

 Wellness Words

Tahini is a sesame seed paste similar in consistency to natural peanut butter. You can find it in most grocery stores in the peanut butter section. If it's not there, try the Middle Eastern section or store.

Black Olive Tapenade

Smoky and salty, this rich spread adds pizzazz to any party.

Yield: 1¼ cup, 10 servings	

Prep time: 2 minutes

Serving size: 2 table-spoons

Each serving has:

40 calories

3 g carbohydrates

4 g fat

0.5 g fiber

0 g protein

2 cups pitted kalamata olives   **1 tsp. garlic powder**

1 TB. vegetable oil   **¼ tsp. crushed red pepper flakes (optional)**

1. In the bowl of a food processor fitted with a metal blade, combine olives, vegetable oil, garlic powder, and crushed red pepper (if using). Pulse for approximately 10 seconds or until you get a blended but textured dip.

2. Serve with thin slices of bread and goat cheese, or as a dip on baked potato chips. Leftover spread will keep in the refrigerator for 3 or 4 days.

Gut Facts

Although black olives have a bit of fat, it is the heart-healthy monounsaturated fat. A rich source of vitamin E too, olives contain disease-fighting antioxidant power.

Bruschetta Spread

You'll adore the blend of garlic and fresh basil in this great spread.

3 medium tomatoes, chopped

½ cup chopped fresh basil

1 tsp. red wine vinegar

1 TB. vegetable oil

½ tsp. garlic powder

¼ tsp. salt

¼ tsp. freshly ground black pepper

Yield: 2 cups, 4 servings
Prep time: 30 minutes
Serving size: ½ cup
Each serving has:
46 calories
4 g carbohydrates
3.5 g fat
1.5 g fiber
0 g protein

1. In a small bowl, combine tomatoes and basil.

2. In another small bowl, combine vinegar, vegetable oil, garlic powder, salt, and pepper. Drizzle oil mixture over tomatoes and basil, and toss gently. Let sit for 20 minutes at room temperature to infuse flavors.

3. Serve with thin rounds of grilled *polenta* for an appetizer or over thinly sliced rounds of French bread.

Wellness Words

Polenta, a cornmeal porridge, is a popular alternative to pasta or rice in northern Italy. You can find precooked polenta in some large grocery stores in the international section. Look for it in a tube shape, precooked and ready to slice and grill Grilled polenta and bruschetta is a wonderful combination.

Strawberry and Balsamic Salsa

Superbly sweet and tangy, this combo is a great complement to chocolate sorbet or salad greens.

Yield: 2 cups, 4 servings
Prep time: 10 minutes
Serving size: ½ cup
Each serving has:
60 calories
10 g carbohydrates
1.5 g fat
1.5 g fiber
0.5 g protein

2 cups strawberries, cleaned, hulled, and chopped fine

2 tsp. sugar

2 TB. freshly squeezed lemon juice (about 1 lemon)

1 tsp. balsamic vinegar

1 tsp. vegetable oil

1. Place strawberries in a medium bowl and set aside.

2. In a small bowl, whisk together sugar, lemon juice, balsamic vinegar, and vegetable oil.

3. Drizzle over strawberries, blending gently to mix. Serve over salad greens or sorbet for dessert.

Digestibles

Balsamic vinegar is known to be rich in phytochemicals linked with a decreased risk of inflammation, heart disease, and cancer. Enjoy it in a salsa like this or as a dressing on your favorite garden salad.

Berry Sweet Salsa

The various berries in this salsa infuse it with a bit of sweet and a tinge of tart.

2 cups mixed berries, frozen and defrosted in refrigerator overnight

¼ cup freshly squeezed lemon juice (about 2 lemons)

1 TB. sugar

Yield: 2 cups, 4 servings
Prep time: 5 minutes plus overnight defrosting time
Serving size: ½ cup
Each serving has:
62 calories
11 g carbohydrates
0 g fat
1.5 g fiber
0.5 g protein

1. In a medium bowl, combine defrosted berries along with any liquid from the defrosting process with lemon juice and sugar.

2. Serve over warm Brownie Bites (recipe in Chapter 21) or over a scoop of your favorite sorbet.

Gut Facts

I enjoy this salsa over chocolate sorbet. The richness of the chocolate with the tangy lemon-berry mixture is so delicious. Berries and chocolate are a great source of disease-fighting anti-oxidants, so feel good about this sweet treat!

Tomato Salsa

This lighter and onion-free version of the favorite Mexican condiment won't trigger your IBS.

Yield: 2 cups, 4 servings
Prep time: 10 minutes
Serving size: ½ cup
Each serving has:
32 calories
5 g carbohydrates
0 g fat
1 g fiber
0 g protein

3 medium tomatoes, chopped

3 TB. freshly squeezed lemon juice or lime juice (about 1 or 2 lemons or 2 or 3 limes)

½ tsp. garlic salt

½ cup chopped fresh cilantro

1. In medium bowl, combine tomatoes, lemon juice, garlic salt, and cilantro.

2. Let sit for about 10 minutes at room temperature to blend ingredients. Serve with tortilla chips.

Digestibles

This salsa is delicious on top of your favorite grilled fish or chicken, too!

Sesame Chicken in Pea Pods

My friend Lisa Kendrick introduced me to this crunchy and savory bite-size crowd-pleasing appetizer.

1 lb. boneless, skinless chicken breasts (about 3 or 4 breasts), cut in bite-size chunks

½ cup oil-based Italian dressing

½ cup sesame seeds

½ cup all-purpose flour

4 TB. vegetable oil

4 cups (loosely packed) snow peas, ends trimmed (½ lb.)

Yield: 45 to 50 pieces, about 12 servings
Prep time: 15 minutes plus 6 hours or overnight marinating time
Cook time: 10 minutes per batch
Serving size: 4 pieces
Each serving has:
185 calories
6 g carbohydrates
9 g fat
2 g fiber
11 g protein

1. In a medium zipper-lock bag or a glass bowl, cover chicken chunks with dressing. Refrigerate overnight to infuse flavor, mixing a few times to ensure chicken is thoroughly coated with dressing.

2. After 6 hours, or the next day, mix sesame seeds and flour in a shallow bowl. Remove chicken from marinade, and discard marinade. Add chicken, a few pieces at a time, to sesame seed mix, pressing down to ensure seeds stick to chicken.

3. Heat a large, nonstick skillet over medium heat. Add 2 tablespoons vegetable oil. Add half of chicken bites to the hot skillet (you'll have to do this in 2 batches). Cook for 5 minutes, turn chicken over, and cook for 5 to 8 more minutes, stirring occasionally, until chicken is cooked through. (Test your largest piece by cutting through to see if it's no longer pink inside and juices are clear, or test with an instant-read thermometer inserted into the center. It should register 160°F.)

4. Remove chicken from the skillet, and place on a paper towel–lined plate to drain.

5. Add remaining 2 tablespoons vegetable oil to the skillet, and cook rest of chicken. Set aside.

6. Fill a medium saucepan ⅔ full of water, and set over high heat. When water is boiling, add snow peas. Cook for 2 minutes. Remove immediately from heat, pour into a colander, and run under cold water to stop the cooking process.

7. To assemble, wrap 1 pea pod around each piece of chicken, and secure with a toothpick. Serve immediately.

 Digestibles

Sometimes I use whole chicken breasts, about 3- or 4-ounce portions, with this same sesame seed and flour mixture. I cook it about 20 minutes longer to ensure it's done. I then slice the chicken into strips and place on top of a garden salad.

Smoked Salmon Pinwheels

The salmon's smoky flavor is complemented nicely by the creamy dill.

Yield: 20 pinwheels, *5 servings*
Prep time: 5 minutes plus 45 minutes chill time
Serving size: 4 pinwheels
Each serving has:
149 calories
3.8 g carbohydrates
9 g fat
0 g fiber
12 g protein

1 (8-oz.) smoked salmon fillet

8 oz. Neufchâtel cheese, or 1 (8-oz.) block light cream cheese, at room temperature

2 TB. finely chopped fresh dill

1. Lay salmon on a piece of wax paper, creating a rectangular shape, approximately 3 inches by 10 inches, overlapping salmon if needed.

2. Spread softened cheese evenly over salmon, and sprinkle with dill.

3. Roll up salmon like a jelly roll so the finished roll is about 10 inches long. Wrap in wax paper, and refrigerate for 45 minutes so the flavors can infuse and cheese firm up.

4. Remove from the refrigerator and slice into ½-inch slices. Serve on top of thinly sliced bread, Melba toast, or thin cucumber rounds.

Gut Facts

Salmon is a well-known source of omega-3 fatty acids, which play a role in both heart health and brain function.

Mini Corn Cakes

These savory morsels are true comfort food in a bite-size package. They're wonderful served alongside warm soup.

1 large egg

½ cup reduced-lactose low-fat milk

2 TB. olive or vegetable oil

½ cup fine-grind cornmeal

¼ cup reduced-fat cheddar cheese, finely grated

½ cup all-purpose flour

½ cup frozen whole kernel corn, defrosted for 20 minutes at room temperature, or fresh corn cut from 1 cob

1½ TB. sugar

½ tsp. garlic powder

¼ tsp. salt

⅛ tsp. cayenne (optional)

1 tsp. baking powder

Yield: 20 corn cakes, 10 servings	
Prep time: 30 minutes	
Cook time: 10 minutes	
Serving size: 2 corn cakes	
Each serving has:	
102 calories	
12 g carbohydrates	
4 g fat	
1 g fiber	
3 g protein	

1. Preheat the oven to 350°F. Spray 24 mini muffin tins with nonstick cooking spray.

2. In a medium bowl, whisk together egg, milk, and oil.

3. Add cornmeal, cheddar cheese, flour, corn, sugar, garlic powder, salt, cayenne (if using), and baking powder, and blend with a spoon.

4. Drop batter by the tablespoonful into the prepared muffin tins. Bake for 8 to 10 minutes. Let sit to cool for about 5 minutes, run a butter knife around the edges of the tins to loosen, remove corn cakes, and serve.

Digestibles

Cornmeal comes in different textures. For this recipe, use the fine grind. It'll make a lighter-textured mini muffin.

Kevin's Mini Beef Kabobs

This is a mini version of a steak house delight, with a noteworthy aromatic herb and mustardy goodness.

Yield: 20 kabobs, 10 servings
Prep time: 20 minutes plus overnight marinating time
Cook time: 10 minutes
Serving size: 2 kabobs
Each serving has:
136 calories
4 g carbohydrates
7 g fat
0.5 g fiber
14 g protein

1 lb. lean steak such as London broil or lean sirloin

⅓ cup vegetable oil

2 TB. red wine vinegar

1 tsp. garlic powder

½ tsp. ground dry mustard

½ tsp. onion salt

2 tsp. dried oregano

20 bamboo skewers, pre-soaked in water

2 cups grape tomatoes (20 tomatoes)

1 large green bell pepper, ribs and seeds removed, and cut into 20 bite-size chunks

1. Cut steak into 40 bite-size chunks and place in a medium nonmetal casserole dish or a large zipper-lock bag.

2. In a small bowl, combine vegetable oil, vinegar, garlic powder, dry mustard, onion salt, and oregano. Drizzle mixture over steak, and toss to coat. Cover with plastic wrap or seal the bag, and refrigerate overnight.

3. The next day, thread steak onto skewers, followed by tomatoes and bell pepper chunks.

4. Grill over hot coals or gas grill for 4 minutes per side until steak is cooked through or until an instant-read thermometer inserted into the center registers 160°F. Serve immediately.

Gut Facts

Lean beef is a great source of the iron your body requires to make the oxygen-carrying protein hemoglobin.

Buffalo Shrimp Bites

A bit tangy and definitely hot, these shrimp bites make a fabulous quick-fix appetizer.

1 lb. extra-large raw frozen shrimp (about 16 to 20 per pound), deveined and deshelled

1 TB. vegetable oil

⅓ **cup hot sauce**

1 TB. butter or trans-fat-free margarine

Yield: 5 servings		
Prep time: 5 minutes		
Cook time: 10 minutes		
Serving size: 4 shrimp		
Each serving has:		
85 calories		
0.5 g carbohydrates		
5.5 g fat		
0 g fiber		
5.6 g protein		

1. In a large skillet over medium heat, combine shrimp and vegetable oil. Cook for about 10 minutes, stirring frequently to ensure even cooking, until shrimp turn pink.

2. Add hot sauce and butter, and stir to coat shrimp.

3. Serve hot with toothpicks.

Digestibles

Make friends with the frozen, deshelled, and deveined shrimp in bags in the frozen section of your grocery store. When you're ready to use the shrimp, defrost it in a colander under cool running water. The shrimp cook in minutes and can be tossed over a salad, pasta, or rice for a quick meal.

Chapter 14

Soups and Salads to Savor

In This Chapter

- Creamy soups to warm your soul
- Jam-packed veggie soups
- Vibrant, wholesome leafy greens
- Delicious salad dressings just a whisk away

Soups are the consummate comfort food; they are warm and delightful on a cold winter's evening. The soups in this chapter range from light and simple to rich and hearty. Enjoy these tasty soups with a garden salad and a crusty roll, and you have a warming, wholesome meal. Or some are a meal unto themselves.

Soups and salads make a wonderful pair. Combine crisp leafy greens with homemade salad dressing, and you'll opt to never buy a bottled version again. Colorful salads add a crunch to your menu while helping you meet your daily veggie quota. As an added bonus, you'll be sure to increase your intake of vitamins A and C and potassium, too.

Simmering Soups

You've gotta love a bowl of hearty stew or a nourishing cup of chicken soup, especially in the winter. And if you're sick? Well, soups are good medicine. Almost everyone loves soup; in fact, if you travel the world you'll find well-known favorites such as minestrone in Italy, gazpacho in Spain, Borscht in Russia, and of course, French onion soup in France.

In this chapter, I did my best to squeeze as many healthy vegetables as I could into each and every soup recipe. After all, that's my job, right? Sipping on steaming soups is a great way to slow down and enjoy your meal. When dining away from home, consider taking some soup to go. Soup packs nicely in a thermos for a quick meal anytime and anywhere!

Super Salads

Lettuce and carrots aren't just "rabbit food." Dark green lettuce is loaded with vitamins and also provides important phytochemicals such as lutein and zeaxanthin, which keep your eyes healthy as they age. These greens contain vitamin K, too, which keeps your bones healthy and your blood clotting properly.

And talk about versatile! Salads can be light for a side dish or a fully loaded complete meal. When making your favorite salad, try to incorporate a vast array of vibrant vegetables all the colors of the rainbow to boost your nutrient intake and keep your body strong.

Pumpkin Soup

Halloween's favorite vegetable makes its way into this sweet and savory soup.

2 (14.5-oz.) cans pumpkin (not pumpkin pie filling)

3½ cups reduced-lactose low-fat milk

¼ cup maple syrup

1 tsp. ground ginger

1 tsp. ground cinnamon

¼ tsp. salt

Yield: 7 cups
Prep time: 5 minutes
Cook time: 15 minutes
Serving size: 1 cup
Each serving has:
123 calories
24 g carbohydrates
1.4 g fat
3.5 g fiber
5.3 g protein

1. In a large saucepan set over medium heat, combine pumpkin, milk, maple syrup, ginger, cinnamon, and salt. Stir for 5 minutes to blend.

2. Reduce heat to low, and allow soup to simmer for 15 minutes to infuse flavors. Remove from heat, and serve with crusty oatmeal or other whole-grain rolls and a colorful side salad.

Gut Facts

Pumpkin is loaded with antioxidants, disease-fighting nutrients associated with lowering risk of macular degeneration, the leading cause of blindness in the elderly.

Butternut Squash Soup with Sage

You'll love this velvety and scrumptious sage-infused soup!

Yield: 6 servings	
Prep time: 20 minutes	
Cook time: 1 to 1½ hours	
Serving size: 1 cup	

Each serving has:

147 calories

22 g carbohydrates

7 g fat

3.6 g fiber

2.5 g protein

3 TB. olive or vegetable oil

2 medium butternut squash, skin on, seeded, and chopped into about 16 large chunks

½ tsp. garlic salt

½ tsp. seasoning salt

¼ tsp. dried sage

2 (14.5-oz.) cans low-sodium fat-free chicken broth

1. Preheat the oven to 350°F. Generously grease the bottom of an 11×15-inch jelly-roll pan with 1 tablespoon olive oil.

2. Place squash flesh side down onto the pan. Sprinkle with garlic salt, seasoning salt, and sage. Drizzle with remaining 2 tablespoons olive oil, and place in oven. Bake for 1 to 1½ hours or until squash is very soft. Remove from the oven, and let cool for 15 minutes.

3. Scoop out flesh of squash, and set aside in a medium bowl. Discard peels.

4. In batches, combine 1 cup broth with 2 cups squash in a blender or a food processor fitted with a metal blade, and purée squash for about 2 minutes per batch or until smooth.

5. Place puréed squash in a stockpot over low heat, add any remaining broth to the pot, and mix to blend. Warm soup to desired temperature and serve.

Digestibles

Butternut squash is a rich source of vitamins A and C. So this is a great soup to keep your immune system healthy!

Basil-Vegetable Soup with Parmesan

Bountiful vegetables are jam-packed into this nourishing soup garnished with lots of fresh chopped basil and freshly grated Parmesan cheese.

3 medium carrots, peeled and sliced into rounds

2 medium celery stalks, chopped

1 (28-oz.) can crushed tomatoes, with juice

1 (14.5-oz.) can low-sodium fat-free chicken broth

¼ tsp. garlic salt

1 tsp. onion powder

1 TB. olive or vegetable oil

1 cup fresh or frozen peas

1 cup fresh basil, chopped into thin strips

1 cup freshly grated Parmesan cheese

Yield: 8 servings
Prep time: 10 minutes
Cook time: 4 to 6 hours
Serving size: 1 cup
Each serving has:
126 calories
12.5 g carbohydrates
5.5 g fat
3.3 g fiber
7 g protein

1. In a slow cooker, combine carrots, celery, tomatoes, chicken broth, garlic salt, onion powder, and olive oil. Set heat to high and cook for 4 hours.

2. Stir in peas. Turn off heat, and let soup sit for 3 to 5 minutes. (If peas are frozen, taste-test prior to serving to ensure they are cooked enough.)

3. Ladle into soup bowls by the cupful, garnish with 2 table-spoons each basil and Parmesan cheese, and serve.

Gut Facts

Muir Glen fire-roasted canned tomatoes are great in this recipe. And although cooking tomatoes lowers the vitamin C content, it actually increases the availability of the tomatoes' lycopene content. Lycopene is an important antioxidant linked with decreasing the risk of cancer and maybe even lowers heart disease risk.

Grandma's Chicken and Rice Soup

Enjoy the lively and fresh tarragon aroma that fills your home from this nourishing soup.

Yield: 16 cups
Prep time: 5 to 10 minutes
Cook time: 20 to 25 minutes
Serving size: 1 cup
Each serving has:
80 calories
7 g carbohydrates
1 g fat
.8 g fiber
10 g protein

1 (14.5-oz.) can diced tomatoes, with juice

2 cups button mushrooms, sliced

1 TB. garlic powder

1 TB. onion powder

$\frac{1}{2}$ tsp. seasoning salt

$1\frac{1}{2}$ tsp. dried tarragon

8 cups low-sodium fat-free chicken broth

3 cups cooked chicken, chopped into bite-size chunks

2 cups cooked brown rice

1. In a large stockpot over high heat, combine tomatoes, mushrooms, garlic powder, onion powder, seasoning salt, tarragon, and chicken broth, and bring to a boil. Reduce heat to low, and simmer for 10 to 15 minutes.

2. Add cooked chicken and rice, simmer for 10 more minutes, and serve.

 Digestibles _____

This is a great soup to make when you have leftover chicken and rice. If you have leftover roasted chicken or store-bought rotisserie chicken, it's perfect for this dish. I keep precooked brown rice in the freezer—it's simple to reheat in this soup.

Thai Chicken and Rice Noodle Soup

Asian-inspired flavors of ginger and sesame permeate in this light soup.

1 TB. vegetable oil

1 TB. fresh or jarred ginger, minced

½ tsp. garlic salt

1 tsp. sesame oil

6 cups reduced-sodium fat-free chicken broth

2 cups button mushrooms, very thinly sliced

1 medium carrot, peeled and cut into thin rounds

3 cups *bok choy* leaves and stalks, finely sliced (1 small head)

2 cups snow peas, ends trimmed and cut in thirds

2 cups diced cooked chicken

2 cups cooked thin rice noodles or rice sticks

¼ cup chopped fresh cilantro or parsley (optional)

Yield: 12 cups
Prep time: 15 minutes
Cook time: 15 to 20 minutes
Serving size: 1 cup
Each serving has:
105 calories
9.4 g carbohydrates
3.4 g fat
1 g fiber
9 g protein

1. In a large stockpot over low heat, combine vegetable oil, ginger, garlic salt, and sesame oil, and heat for 1 minute, stirring frequently.

2. Add chicken broth, mushrooms, carrots, and bok choy, and increase the heat to medium-high. Cook for 10 to 15 minutes or until carrots are fork-tender.

3. Add snow peas, chicken, and noodles, and simmer for 5 more minutes.

4. Remove from heat, ladle into bowls, garnish with cilantro (if using), and serve.

 Wellness Words _____

Bok choy is a member of the brassica family alongside broccoli and kale. Like many other leafy greens, bok choy is a great source of calcium. It resembles a wide stalk of celery with deep green leaves. If you can find baby bok choy, get it. It will be more tender. Bok choy is popular in Asian stir-fry recipes or salad dishes.

Meatball, Barley, and Spinach Soup

This hearty veggie-and-barley soup is protein-packed with tasty, bite-size meatballs.

Yield: 16 cups
Prep time: 35 to 40 minutes
Cook time: 1 hour, 20 minutes
Serving size: 1 cup
Each serving has:
158 calories
12 g carbohydrates
7.4 g fat
2.3 g fiber
10 g protein

1 cup pearled barley	1 TB. plus 1 tsp. onion salt
4 cups low-sodium fat-free chicken broth	½ lb. ground pork
4 cups low-sodium fat-free beef broth	¾ lb. 85-percent-lean ground beef
2 cups water	½ cup grated Parmesan cheese
2 medium carrots, peeled and finely chopped	¼ cup breadcrumbs
2 medium celery stalks, finely chopped	1 TB. Italian seasoning
1 TB. plus 1 tsp. garlic powder	½ tsp. freshly ground black pepper
	1 large egg, beaten
	4 cups fresh baby spinach

Gut Facts

This soup is reminiscent of Italian wedding soup, but instead of pasta, I've used fiber-rich barley. Barley is rich in soluble fiber known for its heart-health benefits and a good fiber choice for those with IBS.

1. In a large stockpot over high heat, combine barley, chicken broth, beef broth, water, carrots, celery, 1 tablespoon garlic powder, and 1 tablespoon onion salt. Bring to rolling boil. Reduce heat to low, and simmer, covered, for 1 hour, 15 minutes.

2. Meanwhile, preheat the oven to 375°F. Spray a nonstick cookie sheet with nonstick cooking spray.

3. In a medium bowl, combine ground pork, beef, Parmesan cheese, breadcrumbs, remaining 1 teaspoon garlic powder, remaining 1 teaspoon onion salt, Italian seasoning, pepper, and egg. Blend meats with seasonings until thoroughly mixed.

4. Roll into small meatballs, about the size of cherry tomatoes, and place on the cookie sheet. Bake meatballs for 7 minutes. Flip meatballs over with a spatula, and cook for 5 or 6 more minutes.

5. Add meatballs and spinach to soup, and simmer for 3 to 5 more minutes or until spinach wilts. Enjoy with crusty rolls for a complete and satisfying meal.

Tasty Beef Stew

This robust beef stew packed with hearty beef and nutritious vegetables will never go out of style.

2 TB. vegetable oil

1 lb. lean stew beef or beef chuck, chopped into bite-size chunks

4 medium carrots, peeled and sliced into thin rounds

4 medium potatoes, skin on, chopped into bite-size chunks

2 cups button mushrooms, sliced

2 (14.5-oz.) cans reduced-sodium fat-free beef broth

3 TB. cornstarch

½ cup reduced-lactose low-fat milk

2 cups frozen peas

Yield: 10 servings
Prep time: 15 minutes
Cook time: 5 hours
Serving size: 1 cup
Each serving has:
235 calories
23 g carbohydrates
8 g fat
3.4 g fiber
17.7 g protein

1. Preheat the oven to 275°F.

2. In a large, nonstick skillet over medium-high heat, combine vegetable oil and beef. Cook for 10 minutes, stirring occasionally, or until meat has browned but is not cooked through.

3. In a 9×13 pan, combine cooked beef, carrots, potatoes, and mushrooms. Set aside.

4. In a medium bowl, whisk together beef broth, cornstarch, and milk. Pour over beef mixture.

5. Cover pan with aluminum foil, and bake for 5 hours.

6. Remove the pan from the oven, add peas, and give a quick stir. Let sit for 5 minutes to quick cook peas before serving with crusty rolls and perhaps the Arugula Salad with Lemon Vinaigrette (recipe later in this chapter).

Gut Facts

Slow, covered cooking keeps the meat tender and moist, unlike higher-heat or dry-cooking methods that can dry a piece of beef.

Bibb Lettuce Salad with Dijon Vinaigrette

The buttery leafy greens in this salad pair beautifully with the mustardy light dressing.

Yield: 4 servings
Prep time: 10 minutes
Serving size: 1 cup
Each serving has:
137 calories
3 g carbohydrates
13.5 g fat
1.2 g fiber
1 g protein

2 medium heads *Bibb lettuce*, **rinsed and torn into small pieces**

1 cup cherry or grape tomatoes, cut in half

1 TB. white wine vinegar

1 tsp. Dijon mustard

$\frac{1}{4}$ tsp. garlic salt

$\frac{1}{4}$ tsp. freshly ground black pepper

$\frac{1}{4}$ cup extra-virgin olive oil

1. In a salad bowl, place lettuce and top with tomatoes. Set aside.

2. In a small bowl, whisk together vinegar, Dijon mustard, garlic salt, pepper, and extra-virgin olive oil.

3. Drizzle dressing evenly over salad, and gently mix. You could serve with Dry-Rubbed Grilled Tuna (recipe in Chapter 16) and Kasha Pilaf (recipe in Chapter 20).

Wellness Words

Bibb lettuce is a member of the butter head lettuce family. A pale green, buttery soft leaf makes this lettuce a prized treat. You'll find a bit of potassium and vitamin A in this leafy vegetable with only 3 calories per leaf.

Arugula Salad with Lemon Vinaigrette

The peppery green *arugula* makes a nice complement to the citrus dressing in this surprising salad.

4 cups baby arugula	$\frac{1}{4}$ **tsp. salt**
2 TB. freshly squeezed lemon juice (1 lemon)	$\frac{1}{4}$ **tsp. freshly ground black pepper**
$\frac{1}{4}$ **cup extra-virgin olive or vegetable oil**	$\frac{1}{2}$ **cup flaked Parmesan cheese**

Yield: 4 servings
Prep time: 5 minutes
Serving size: 1 cup
Each serving has:
169 calories
1.3 g carbohydrates
16 g fat
trace fiber
4 g protein

1. Place arugula in a salad bowl, and set aside.

2. In a small bowl, whisk together lemon juice, extra-virgin olive oil, salt, and pepper.

3. Drizzle over arugula, toss to blend, and sprinkle with Parmesan cheese.

Variation: Enjoy this salad as is, or get creative and add some garden veggies, toasted walnuts, or grilled chicken.

 Wellness Words

> **Arugula** is a fragrant and peppery green leafy vegetable popular in Italian cuisine. It's fabulous as a salad green but just as nice made into pesto, topped on pizza, or sautéed with a bit of olive oil and served wilted like spinach. You can use regular arugula for this recipe, but do try to get baby arugula, which is extra tender.

Confetti Rice Salad

This colorful salad has a nutty taste that pairs well with an Asian-style dressing.

Yield: 7 servings
Prep time: 10 minutes
Serving size: 1 cup
Each serving has:
184 calories
25.5 g carbohydrates
7 g fat
3 g fiber
5 g protein

2 TB. Asian chili sauce

2 TB. reduced-sodium tamari or soy sauce

1 TB. rice wine vinegar

1 TB. sesame oil

2 TB. olive or vegetable oil

1½ cups *forbidden rice*, cooked

1½ cups jasmine rice, cooked

1 medium red bell pepper, ribs and seeds removed, and chopped into bite-size chunks

1 medium yellow bell pepper, ribs and seeds removed, and chopped into bite-size chunks

2 medium carrots, peeled and cut into thin rounds

1 cup shelled *edamame*

1. In a large serving dish, whisk together chili sauce, tamari, rice wine vinegar, sesame oil, and olive oil.

2. Stir in forbidden rice, jasmine rice, red bell pepper, yellow bell pepper, carrots, and edamame. Serve immediately, or refrigerate for at least 1 hour for a cold salad option.

Wellness Words

Forbidden rice is a medium Chinese black rice that's actually dark purple. It cooks up in 30 minutes and is nutty and delicious. You can often find forbidden rice in health food stores or in the international sections of large grocery stores. Its purple color is from the phytochemical anthocyanins, which are linked with lowering heart disease risk. When cooking rice, keep in mind its volume triples after cooking. Edamame are immature soybeans and do contain FODMAPs, so don't overdo it! They are often available frozen. If using frozen, defrost prior to use.

German Potato Salad

A favorite in my home during the holidays, this hand-me-down salad from my German grandma is truly *dill*-icious!

9 medium red-skinned potatoes, skin on and scrubbed

¼ cup apple cider vinegar, or more to taste

¼ cup vegetable oil, or more to taste

½ tsp. onion salt

1 or 2 extra-large dill pickles, cut into bite-size chunks

2 TB. chopped fresh parsley

Yield: 10 servings
Prep time: 15 minutes
Cook time: 20 minutes
Serving size: ½ cup
Each serving has:
167 calories
29 g carbohydrates
5 g fat
3 g fiber
2 g protein

1. In an extra-large stockpot over high heat, add potatoes and just enough water to cover them. Bring to a boil, and cook for 20 minutes or until fork-tender.

2. Remove from heat and place potatoes in a colander. Rinse with cold water until they're cool enough you can handle them.

3. Peel potatoes with a vegetable peeler or a paring knife, cut into chunks, and place in a large bowl. (You may want to peel under cold running water because they may be still hot.)

4. Drizzle potatoes with vinegar and gently mix. Stir in vegetable oil, onion salt, pickles, and parsley. Refrigerate overnight.

5. The next day, stir potatoes. Leave at room temperature for 1 hour prior to serving. Add more vinegar or oil if you like.

Variation: If you can't find big dill pickles at your grocery's deli counter, substitute 5 or 6 dill spears instead.

 Gut Facts

Potatoes have gotten a bad rap. Thought to be heavy in calories and low in nutritional content, a small potato has about 130 calories, 3 grams fiber, and 3 grams protein. Potatoes are a great source of potassium and vitamin C, too!

Carrot Salad with Cranberries and Orange

My sister, Trisha, ordered this refreshingly sweet and crisp salad in Bartlett's Farm on Nantucket, where we took a pit stop while biking to the beach. This is my tweaked version so it's easier on the tummy.

Yield: 6 servings
Prep time: 10 minutes plus 2 hours chill time
Serving size: ½ cup
Each serving has:
172 calories
21 g carbohydrates
9 g fat
3 g fiber
2 g protein

1 (10-oz.) bag shredded carrots or about 6 carrots, peeled and grated

⅔ cup dried cranberries, chopped

½ cup walnuts, chopped

1 TB. maple syrup

¼ cup reduced-fat mayonnaise

1½ tsp. red wine vinegar

2 tsp. orange zest

1. In a large bowl, combine carrots, cranberries, and walnuts.

2. In a small bowl, whisk together maple syrup, mayonnaise, red wine vinegar, and orange zest.

3. Drizzle dressing over carrot mixture, and refrigerate for 2 hours. Enjoy with grilled fish and a baked potato.

Gut Facts

Walnuts are a great source of omega-3 fats, a heart-healthy fat. Walnuts also contain vitamin E, magnesium, B vitamins, and fiber.

Strawberry Romaine Salad with Poppy Seed Dressing

The specialty of this recipe is the homemade creamy dressing and the fresh fruit.

1 large head romaine lettuce, chopped

2 cups fresh strawberries, hulled and chopped

2 kiwifruit, peeled and sliced into thin rounds

¼ cup reduced-fat mayonnaise

1 TB. red wine vinegar

2 TB. sugar

2 TB. reduced-lactose low-fat milk

1 TB. poppy seeds

Yield: 5 servings		
Prep time: 15 minutes		
Serving size: approximately 1 cup		
Each serving has:		
113 calories		
19 g carbohydrates		
4 g fat		
4.6 g fiber		
2 g protein		

1. In a medium or large salad bowl, add lettuce. Top with strawberries followed by kiwifruit.

2. In a glass jar, combine mayonnaise, red wine vinegar, sugar, milk, and poppy seeds. Cover the jar tightly, and shake well.

3. Drizzle dressing over salad, and serve. Refrigerate any leftover dressing for a day or two.

 Digestibles

For a protein-rich meal, try adding grilled steak or chicken on top of this sweet salad.

Baby Spinach and Orange Drizzle

Tender leafy greens are a great match for this tangy and light dressing.

Yield: 4 servings
Prep time: 10 minutes
Serving size: 1 cup
Each serving has:
231 calories
13 g carbohydrates
19 g fat
2.8 g fiber
4 g protein

4 cups baby spinach, washed

1 (11-oz.) can mandarin orange segments, drained and rinsed

½ cup sliced almonds

¼ cup olive or vegetable oil

2 TB. orange juice

2 tsp. red wine vinegar

1 TB. maple syrup

½ tsp. salt

¼ tsp. freshly ground black pepper

1. In a medium salad bowl, add washed spinach. Layer orange segments and almonds on top.

2. In a small bowl, whisk together olive oil, orange juice, red wine vinegar, maple syrup, salt, and pepper.

3. Drizzle dressing over salad, and serve.

Gut Facts

Almonds add a nice crunch to this sweet salad. They're also a rich source of heart-healthy monounsaturated fats and magnesium.

15

Scrumptious Sandwiches

In This Chapter

- ◆ Light lunch pitas
- ◆ Fabulous, quick-fix veggie sandwiches
- ◆ Filling, fiber-rich wraps
- ◆ Belly-good beefy dips

For lunch or for an alternative to a large meal, sandwiches definitely fit the bill. Sandwiches were my mom's favorite solution for easy, crowd-pleasing lunchtime nosh—and she had a crowd to feed with nine kids! Filling your sandwich with a variety of tasty and well-tolerated vegetables and lean protein sources can be a great start to a light meal.

Instead of heading straight for the vending machine or nearest fast-food restaurant, create one of the great sandwich selections found in this chapter for a pack-along lunch. Say good-bye to the fast-food fat fest, and note how energized you feel after eating one of these awesome assortments instead. Taking a few moments to whip up one of these yummy creations will make your taste buds and tummy more than happy!

Slam Burgers in Pitas

A favorite back in my college days, this cheesy meat is easy to make and tasty to eat!

Yield: 4 sandwiches
Prep time: 5 minutes
Cook time: 10 to 13 minutes
Serving size: 1 sandwich
Each serving has:
394 calories
16 g carbohydrates
24 g fat
3 g fiber
31 g protein

1 lb. 85-percent-lean ground beef

½ tsp. onion powder

½ tsp. garlic salt

1 cup reduced-fat cheddar cheese, grated

4 small whole-wheat pita pockets

8 leaves lettuce

1 medium tomato, sliced into 8 slices

Dill pickle slices (optional)

1. Spray a large, nonstick skillet with nonstick cooking spray and set over medium heat. Add ground beef, and cook, stirring, for 8 to 10 minutes. Drain any excess fat from meat.

2. Sprinkle meat with onion powder, garlic salt, and cheese, and mix to blend. Cook for 2 or 3 more minutes or until cheese is completely melted and beef is thoroughly cooked. Remove from heat.

3. Trim tops of pita pockets to create openings, and spoon meat evenly among pita pockets. Add lettuce, tomato slices, and a few slices of pickle (if using) to each pita, and serve.

 Digestibles

For a wheat-free alternative, try spreading the meat mixture inside a warmed brown rice tortilla and roll up burrito-style!

Toasted Cheese, Avocado, and Tomato Pitas

Creamy and gooey all in one bite, this pita sandwich is my friend Sophie's favorite!

4 small whole-wheat pita pockets

4 slices sharp cheddar cheese (deli sliced or prepackaged cheddar slices)

½ medium avocado, sliced in 8 thin slices

1 medium tomato, sliced in 8 slices

Yield: 4 sandwiches
Prep time: 5 to 10 minutes
Cook time: 2 to 5 minutes
Serving size: 1 sandwich
Each serving has:
248 calories
19.5 g carbohydrates
14 g fat
5 g fiber
11 g protein

1. Trim tops of pita pockets to create openings.

2. Add 1 slice cheddar inside each pita pocket, followed by 2 avocado slices, and 2 tomato slices.

3. Place pitas in a toaster oven for about 3 minutes to melt cheese or microwave on high for 45 to 55 seconds or until cheese is melted. This sandwich is perfect paired with a bowl of tomato soup.

Variation: For a **Hearty Toasted Veggie and Cheese Pitas,** sauté mushrooms, zucchini slices, or summer squash rounds in a skillet with olive or vegetable oil until browned and add to pita.

Gut Facts

Avocados are rich in monounsaturated fats, the heart-healthy fats. To choose a ripe avocado, pick one that has a small amount of give to it—not too firm and not too squishy!

Outrageous Mushroom Melt

This creamy, earthy sandwich will melt in your mouth!

Yield: 2 sandwiches
Prep time: 5 minutes
Cook time: 5 to 10 minutes
Serving size: 1 sandwich
Each serving has:
268 calories
31 g carbohydrates
10 g fat
5.5 g fiber
17 g protein

1 TB. olive or vegetable oil

1 cup button mushrooms, sliced

1 cup baby portobello (crimini) mushrooms, sliced

½ tsp. garlic powder

2 slices reduced-fat Swiss cheese

2 whole-grain English muffins, cut in half

2 slices tomato

1. In a medium skillet over medium heat, add olive oil, button mushrooms, baby portobello mushrooms, and garlic powder. Cook, stirring, for about 5 to 10 minutes or until mushrooms are browned and soft. Drain any extra liquid from pan.

2. Place Swiss cheese over hot mushrooms. Remove skillet from heat, and set aside to allow cheese to melt.

3. Meanwhile, toast English muffins.

4. Using a spatula, divide mushroom-cheese mixture evenly and place atop 2 English muffin halves. Add 1 tomato slice, and top with remaining English muffin halves. Enjoy with baked potato chips and a handful of baby carrots or a warm bowl of Pumpkin Soup (recipe in Chapter 14).

Gut Facts

Reduced-fat Swiss cheese comes in varying fat content, so be sure to check the labels or ask for nutrition facts information. Jarlsberg lite is one of my lower-fat favorites.

Smoked Gouda, Bacon, and Spinach Wraps

Smoky and savory flavors infuse the green leafy veggies in this winning wrap.

4 (8- to 10-in.) whole-wheat tortillas

8 slices turkey bacon, cooked

1 cup grated smoked Gouda cheese

8 to 12 sun-dried tomato halves

2 cups fresh raw baby spinach, well washed and dried

Yield: 4 sandwiches
Prep time: 5 to 10 minutes
Cook time: 3 to 5 minutes
Serving size: 1 sandwich
Each serving has:
304 calories
22 g carbohydrates
11 g fat
3 g fiber
14 g protein

1. Preheat the oven to 350°F.

2. On a cookie sheet, arrange tortillas in a single layer. Top each with 2 slices bacon, ¼ cup Gouda cheese, and 2 or 3 sun-dried tomatoes. Bake for 3 to 5 minutes or until cheese melts.

3. Top each tortilla with ½ cup raw spinach leaves, and roll up tortillas. Enjoy this light sandwich with a cup of your favorite soup.

Gut Facts

You can find sun-dried tomatoes in the produce section of most grocery stores. These sweet and tangy tomatoes add a nice touch to this flavorful sandwich and are a great source of lycopene, the phytochemical with cancer-protection properties.

Lemony Tuna Salad Wraps with Fresh Dill

This light, herb-infused tuna salad wrap is perfect for a quick-fix anytime meal.

Yield: 4 sandwiches
Prep time: 5 to 10 minutes
Serving size: 1 sandwich
Each serving has:
242 calories
23 g carbohydrates
9 g fat
3.5 g fiber
16 g protein

2 (5-oz.) cans albacore or chunk light tuna (packed in water), drained and rinsed

$\frac{1}{4}$ cup reduced-fat mayonnaise

2 TB. freshly squeezed lemon juice (about 1 lemon)

1 medium celery stalk, finely chopped

$\frac{1}{2}$ tsp. onion powder

1 tsp. chopped fresh dill

4 (8- to 10-in.) whole-grain tortillas

1 cup chopped lettuce

1 cup grated carrots

1. In a small bowl, combine tuna, mayonnaise, lemon juice, celery, onion powder, and dill. Mix with a fork to blend.

2. Divide tuna salad evenly among 4 tortillas. Top each with $\frac{1}{4}$ cup chopped lettuce and $\frac{1}{4}$ cup grated carrots. Roll up tortilla, and enjoy with Basil-Vegetable Soup with Parmesan (recipe in Chapter 14).

Digestibles

Canned tuna is high in added sodium, similar to other canned food products. To reduce the sodium content, which is often more than 300 milligrams sodium per (5-ounce) can, rinse the tuna in a colander under running water before adding to a recipe.

Open-Face French Dip

This mouthwatering and juicy sandwich is a meat lover's dream come true.

1 TB. olive oil

½ small yellow onion, chopped in large chunks

2 cloves garlic, sliced in half

1 (14.5-oz.) can reduced-sodium fat-free beef broth

1 tsp. fresh thyme, whole leaves only

1 small (12-in.) crusty baguette

2 tsp. butter, at room temperature (optional)

4 slices roast beef (deli or leftovers, about ⅓ lb.)

Yield: 2 sandwiches
Prep time: 5 to 10 minutes
Cook time: 5 to 8 minutes
Serving size: 1 sandwich
Each serving has:
431 calories
54 g carbohydrates
11.3 g fat
2 g fiber
27 g protein

1. In a medium skillet over medium heat, combine olive oil, onion, and garlic. Sauté for 2 or 3 minutes or until onion wilts and garlic infuses oil. Remove and discard garlic.

2. Slowly add beef broth and thyme to the skillet, reduce heat to medium-low, and simmer for 2 minutes. Remove from heat, remove and discard onion, and set skillet aside.

3. Preheat the broiler to high.

4. Cut baguette in half lengthwise and place cut side up on a cookie sheet. Spread each baguette half evenly with butter (if using). Toast under the broiler for about 1 or 2 minutes or until lightly browned. Watch carefully to avoid burning. Remove and cut each bread slice in half to make 4 pieces.

5. Add roast beef slices to broth mixture, and submerse in broth for 5 seconds to quickly warm meat.

6. Using tongs, remove 1 slice beef and place on top of each baguette.

7. To serve, place a small ramekin or custard cup of broth mixture on a plate with 2 half sandwiches. Dip sandwich into broth (*au jus*), or drizzle broth onto the sandwich, and enjoy, perhaps alongside Bibb Lettuce Salad with Dijon Vinaigrette (recipe in Chapter 14).

Gut Facts

Au jus is French for "with juice" and refers to a food that's served in natural juices or gravy.

Chapter 16

Surf and Turf

In This Chapter

- ◆ Sensational shellfish
- ◆ Fantastic fish dishes
- ◆ Sizzling steak recipes
- ◆ Beefy comfort foods

Hearty, protein-rich meals help keep your belly full and your muscles strong. From water to land, you can enjoy all these delectable flavors while still feeling your very best. In this chapter, you discover new dinner-party-worthy recipes such as Sautéed Italian-Style Shrimp or Sirloin Skewers to downright comfort foods including Irish Shepherd's Pie.

There's no room for boredom in this chapter. A wide range of recipes are yours for the taking. Enjoy the many tender beef choices or succulent seafood selections that are naturally nourishing and pleasing to your palate.

Recipes from the Sea

You can't go wrong when adding brain food to your diet. Experts have found that people who eat at least one fish meal a week are less likely to develop Alzheimer's disease when compared with those who never consume our seafaring friends. In addition, the American Heart Association recommends two fish meals per week to help your cardiovascular system stay healthy, too. Fish with a naturally higher fat content such as salmon, mackerel, and tuna are your best bets when it comes to providing omega-3 fats, the good fats associated with lowering risk of heart attack and stroke.

Many seafood selections are naturally low in total fat, including sole, halibut, and shrimp, and they're also a great source of complete protein. Fish is nutrient-rich, and provides a good dose of calcium, phosphorus, iron, zinc, iodine, and magnesium.

The Best of Beef

The flavorful beefy dishes in this chapter have been carefully designed with your IBS body in mind. Lean beef is a great source of protein, iron, and B vitamins. When you serve these tasty meats, your family *won't* be asking, "Where's the beef?"

Because beef typically has more overall fat and saturated fat than most poultry and fish options, don't overdo the portion sizes of your beefy favorites. Select lean choices such as round, sirloin, chuck, and loin. Buy "choice" or "select" grades versus "prime," which tends to contain more fat. Purchase extra-lean ground beef, or 90-percent-lean for multi-ingredient dishes, and allow a bit more fat for flavor for burgers, say in the 85-percent-lean range.

Tasty Vietnamese Shrimp Curry

There's lots to love in this seafood dish spiced with curry to really emphasize the Southeast Asian flavors.

1 TB. *peanut oil*

1 tsp. sesame oil

1 lb. (16 to 20) extra-large raw shrimp, peeled and deveined

1 tsp. garlic powder

1 TB. minced ginger

1 TB. firmly packed brown sugar

1 TB. curry powder

½ cup low-sodium fat-free chicken broth

2 TB. reduced-sodium tamari

1 large potato, baked, peeled, and chopped into large chunks

Yields: 4 servings
Prep time: 5 minutes
Cook time: 16 minutes
Serving size: 4 or 5 shrimp
Each serving has:
218 calories
16 g carbohydrates
6.5 g fat
trace fiber
23 g protein

1. In a large skillet over medium heat, combine peanut oil, sesame oil, and shrimp. Sauté for 5 to 8 minutes or until shrimp is fully pink. Remove shrimp and set aside.

2. Add garlic powder, ginger, brown sugar, and curry powder to the skillet, and mix to blend. Reduce heat to low, and slowly add chicken broth and tamari. Simmer for 5 minutes.

3. Add chunks of potato, and return shrimp to the skillet. Cook for 2 or 3 more minutes. Serve with brown rice and steamed green beans.

 Wellness Words _____

Peanut oil is pale yellow oil with a nutty flavor. Peanut oil has a high smoking point, which means it can be heated to high temperatures without smoking.

Sautéed Italian-Style Shrimp

A tasty blend of herbs and garlic infuses this easy shellfish dish.

Yield: 4 servings
Prep time: 10 minutes
Cook time: 8 minutes
Serving size: 4 or 5 shrimp
Each serving has:
180 calories
1 g carbohydrates
9.5 g fat
0 g fiber
22.5 g protein

2 TB. olive or vegetable oil

1 lb. (16 to 20) extra-large raw shrimp, peeled and deveined

1 tsp. garlic powder

1 tsp. onion salt

¼ cup chopped fresh basil

¼ cup chopped fresh parsley

1. In a large skillet over medium heat, combine olive oil and shrimp. Sauté for 5 to 8 minutes or until shrimp is fully pink.

2. Sprinkle shrimp with garlic powder, onion salt, basil, and parsley, and mix to blend. Remove from heat.

3. Serve over rice and alongside Bibb Lettuce Salad with Dijon Vinaigrette (recipe in Chapter 14).

Digestibles

For a great quick-fix meal, use frozen shrimp that's been peeled and deveined. Keep some in your freezer and cook as a topping on pasta, over rice, or on top of salad greens.

Dry-Rubbed Grilled Tuna

Lots of herbs and spices kick this tuna into the all-star category!

1 (1-lb.) tuna steaks

2 TB. paprika

2 tsp. ground thyme

2 tsp. dried basil

2 tsp. garlic salt

1 tsp. onion powder

½ tsp. freshly ground black pepper

Dash cayenne (optional)

Yield: 4 servings
Prep time: 5 minutes
Cook time: 8 to 10 minutes
Serving size: 1 piece (¼ tuna steak)
Each serving has:
92 calories
0 g carbohydrates
1 g fat
0 g fiber
20 g protein

1. Preheat the grill.

2. Lay tuna steak on a large plate.

3. In a small bowl, combine paprika, thyme, basil, garlic salt, onion powder, pepper, and cayenne (if using).

4. Gently rub ½ of spices into one side of tuna, evenly covering in a thin layer. Flip over tuna, and rub remaining spices on the other side.

5. Place tuna on grill, and cook for 4 minutes. Flip over tuna, and cook for 3 or 4 more minutes or until cooked through. Divide steak into 4 even portions, and serve immediately.

 Gut Facts

Tuna is rich in omega-3 fatty acids, the fats associated with lowering risk of heart disease and stroke.

Seared Sea Scallops

These seaworthy delights almost melt in your mouth with just a hint of salt, pepper, and thyme.

Yield: *4 servings*
Prep time: 5 minutes
Cook time: 3 minutes
Serving size: 4 scallops
Each serving has:
99 calories
0 g carbohydrates
6 g fat
0 g fiber
10 g protein

1 to 1¼ lb. (16) sea scallops

1 TB. olive oil

2 tsp. butter

¾ tsp. salt

1 tsp. freshly ground black pepper

½ tsp. ground thyme

1. Rinse scallops with water, and pat dry with paper towels. Trim muscle on side of scallop.

2. In a medium skillet over medium heat, combine olive oil and butter.

3. In a small bowl, combine salt, pepper, and thyme. Sprinkle ½ of herb mixture over one side of scallops.

4. Place scallops salted side down in the skillet. Season the other side of scallops with remaining salt mixture.

5. Cook scallops for about 1½ minutes. Flip over scallops, and cook for 1½ more minutes. Be sure scallops are no longer pink and are fully opaque. Serve on top of arugula salad or with the Farmer's Market Pasta Salad (recipe in Chapter 18).

Gut Facts

Sea scallops are the larger scallops, and bay scallops are the smaller, bite-size scallops.

Heavenly Halibut

Light and lemony make this fish simply wonderful.

2 TB. olive or vegetable oil

2 TB. lemon juice (1 lemon)

$\frac{1}{2}$ tsp. dried basil

1 tsp. fresh or jarred ginger, minced

$\frac{1}{2}$ tsp. onion salt

$\frac{1}{4}$ tsp. freshly ground black pepper

2 (8-oz.) halibut fillets, skinned

Yield: 4 servings
Prep time: 5 minutes
Cook time: 10 minutes
Serving size: 1 piece (about $\frac{1}{2}$ fillet)
Each serving has:
183 calories
0 g carbohydrates
9.5 g fat
0 g fiber
23 g protein

1. Preheat the oven to 400°F.

2. In a small bowl, whisk together olive oil, lemon juice, basil, ginger, onion salt, and pepper.

3. Place halibut on a nonstick cookie sheet and evenly coat with lemon-ginger mixture.

4. Bake on the middle rack for 10 minutes or until halibut is cooked through and flakes easily with a fork. Cut each fillet into 2 even portions, and enjoy with the Arugula Salad with Lemon Vinaigrette (recipe in Chapter 14).

Gut Facts

Halibut is a type of flat fish whose light flavor is easily complemented by a variety of flavors. Halibut is easy to over-cook, so keep a close eye on it as it cooks to ensure a moist piece of fish.

Patrick's Famous Quick-Fix Salmon

Super-moist with a hint of tangy sweetness, this salmon is your best quick-fix fish ever!

Yield: 4 servings
Prep time: 5 to 10 minutes
Cook time: 7 minutes
Serving size: 1 piece
Each serving has:
292 calories
3 g carbohydrates
21 g fat
0 g fiber
22 g protein

1 (1-lb.) salmon fillet

1 TB. sugar

¼ tsp. onion salt

¼ cup olive or vegetable oil

½ tsp. dry mustard

2 TB. red wine vinegar

1 tsp. poppy seeds

1. Place salmon on a microwave-safe dish.

2. In a small bowl, mix sugar, onion salt, olive oil, dry mustard, red wine vinegar, and poppy seeds. Drizzle evenly over salmon.

3. Cover salmon with a paper towel, and microwave for 7 minutes or until thoroughly cooked. Cut into 4 even pieces, and serve immediately.

Gut Facts

Salmon is one of the best sources of heart-healthy omega-3 fats. You can buy salmon wild or farm-raised. Because farm-raised salmon generally contains more polychlorinated biphenyls (PCBs), likely derived from the fishmeal they are commonly fed, try to choose wild salmon when it's available. PCBs have been banned since 1977 because they're linked to risk of cancer and negatively impact reproductive health.

Sole Sauté

This delightful fish dish has a tangy zip and citrus infusion.

¾ cup all-purpose flour

1 tsp. onion salt

½ tsp. freshly ground black pepper

4 (about ¼-lb.) fresh sole fillets

2 TB. olive or vegetable oil

2 TB. chopped fresh parsley

1 TB. butter

2 TB. freshly squeezed lemon juice (1 lemon)

2 TB. brined capers

Yield: 4 servings
Prep time: 5 to 10 minutes
Cook time: 5 minutes
Serving size: 1 piece
Each serving has:
273 calories
18 g carbohydrates
11 g fat
.7 g fiber
24 g protein

1. In a medium, shallow bowl, combine flour, onion salt, and pepper. Dip sole into flour to give a light dusting.

2. In a large, nonstick skillet over medium-high heat, add olive oil. When oil is hot, add sole and cook for 2 minutes per side.

3. Add parsley, butter, lemon juice, and capers, and stir to melt butter and disperse ingredients. Simmer for 1 more minute. Enjoy with a side of rice and Glazed Carrots (recipe in Chapter 19).

Gut Facts

Capers are pickled flower buds that offer a tangy flavor to a dish, especially Mediterranean fare. Find brined capers in the pickle and olive section of your grocery store.

Creamy Tuna Casserole with Peas

If you're a fan of tuna melts, this creamy, garlic-infused dish is for you!

Yield: 6 servings
Prep time: 20 to 30 minutes
Cook time: 25 to 30 minutes
Serving size: ⅙ casserole
Each serving has:
388 calories
47 g carbohydrates
14 g fat
3 g fiber
19 g protein

½ lb. whole-wheat penne or other short pasta

2 (5-oz.) cans solid white albacore tuna, packed in water, drained

1 cup frozen peas

4 TB. olive or vegetable oil

1 TB. butter or trans-fat-free margarine

¼ cup all-purpose flour

½ tsp. garlic salt

2 cups reduced-lactose low-fat milk

½ cup whole-wheat or gluten-free Italian bread-crumbs

2 TB. chopped fresh parsley

1. Preheat the oven to 350°F. Spray a 9×13 pan with nonstick cooking spray.

2. Cook pasta according to package directions. Drain and rinse pasta in a colander, and place in the 9×13 pan.

3. Top pasta with tuna followed by peas. Set aside.

4. In a medium saucepan over medium heat, combine 2 table-spoons olive oil and butter, and heat until butter is melted. Stir in flour and garlic salt. Increase heat to medium-high, and slowly pour in milk, whisking to blend. Continue to stir, and this will form a creamy sauce in about 2 or 3 minutes. Remove from heat.

5. Pour creamy sauce over pasta-tuna mixture, and gently stir to combine.

6. In a small bowl, combine breadcrumbs and remaining 2 tablespoons olive oil. Sprinkle evenly over tuna mixture, covering casserole. Bake for 20 to 25 minutes or until bubbling. Remove from the oven, garnish with parsley, and serve.

Digestibles

To eliminate the fructans in this comfort food dish, you can substitute rice, corn, or quinoa pasta for the wheat pasta. The majority of lactose has been removed from this recipe to keep your belly at ease.

Marinated Flank Steak with Soy Sauce and Shallots

Full of flavor, this savory steak with a hint of citrus is absolutely delectable.

1 lb. flank steak	**1 shallot, cut into large chunks**
½ cup freshly squeezed lemon juice	**1 tsp. dried basil**
⅓ cup reduced-sodium tamari or soy sauce	**1 tsp. garlic powder**

> *Yields: 4 servings*
>
> **Prep time:** 5 minutes plus overnight marinate time
>
> **Cook time:** 12 to 16 minutes
>
> **Serving size:** 1 piece
>
> **Each serving has:**
>
> 249 calories
>
> 1.5 g carbohydrates
>
> 12 g fat
>
> 0 g fiber
>
> 32 g protein

1. Place flank steak in a large zipper-lock bag.

2. Add lemon juice, tamari, shallots, basil, and garlic powder. Close the bag, and give it a good shake to mix. Place the bag in the refrigerator to marinate overnight.

3. The next day, preheat the grill.

4. Remove steak from the zipper-lock bag, discarding any shallots that adhere to meat. Discard the marinade. Place steak on the hot grill, and cook for 6 to 8 minutes per side.

5. Remove steak from the grill and cut meat into 4 even pieces. To cut flank steak, it is best to cut across the grain into thin strips. You might enjoy this dish with Sweet Potato Fries and Peppers and Mushroom Medley (recipes in Chapter 19).

Digestibles

Some meat is more tender when you cut it across the grain. This means you cut the meat perpendicular to the direction of the meat fibers.

Burgers to Beat the Band

You'll enjoy these mouthwatering all-American herb-infused burgers. But don't forget the golden rule of perfectly grilled burgers: only flip once!

Yield: 4 burgers	
Prep time: 10 minutes	
Cook time: 14 minutes	
Serving size: 1 burger	
Each serving has:	
311 calories	
10 g carbohydrates	
19 g fat	
.6 g fiber	
24 g protein	

1 lb. 85-percent-lean beef

½ cup plain, whole-wheat, or gluten-free breadcrumbs

1 large egg

1 TB. chopped fresh thyme

1 TB. chopped fresh rosemary

1 tsp. onion salt

1. Preheat the grill.

2. In a large mixing bowl, combine beef, breadcrumbs, egg, thyme, rosemary, and onion salt. Using clean hands, mix well.

3. Form into 4 burger patties, each about ½ to ¾ inch thick.

4. Grill burgers for 7 minutes, flip over, and cook for 7 more minutes or until an instant-read thermometer inserted into the center registers 160°F.

Digestibles

Ground beef comes in different varieties depending on the fat content. Because the fat in beef is rich in saturated fat, the fat linked with heart disease, opt for the leaner varieties like 85 to 90 percent lean when possible. Ground chicken and turkey breast are lean options you can substitute for ground beef in your favorite recipes.

Sirloin Skewers

The wonderfully tangy beef makes this vegetable-rich main entrée a nutritional winner.

1 lb. sirloin, cut into bite-size chunks

½ cup olive or vegetable oil

3 TB. red wine vinegar

1 tsp. garlic salt

2 TB. Italian seasoning

1 TB. Dijon mustard

1 green bell pepper, ribs and seeds removed, and cut into bite-size chunks

2 cups button mushrooms

2 cups cherry tomatoes

8 to 10 large bamboo skewers, soaked in water

Yield: 4 servings
Prep time: 15 to 20 minutes plus 6 hours or overnight marinate time
Cook time: 10 to 15 minutes
Serving size: 2 skewers
Each serving has:
369 calories
6 g carbohydrates
26.5 g fat
2 g fiber
26 g protein

1. In a large zipper-lock bag, combine sirloin, olive oil, red wine vinegar, garlic salt, Italian seasoning, and Dijon mustard. Close the bag, and give it a good shake to mix. Place the bag in the refrigerator to marinate for 6 hours or overnight.

2. When meat is finished marinating, preheat the grill.

3. Remove sirloin from the bag, discard marinade, and thread onto the skewers, alternating meat with green bell pepper chunks, mushrooms, and tomatoes.

4. Place skewers on the grill, and cook, rotating every 5 minutes, for about 2 or 3 rotations, or until an instant-read thermometer inserted into the center registers 160°F.

 Digestibles

Adding colorful vegetables to these skewers encourages your diners to eat more veggies and less meat!

Curried Beef and Broccoli

Aromatic curry and fragrant ginger infuse the beef in this tasty dish.

Yield: 4 servings
Prep time: 10 minutes
Cook time: 10 to 15 minutes
Serving size: 1½ cups
Each serving has:
322 calories
9 g carbohydrates
17 g fat
1.5 g fiber
33 g protein

1 lb. flank steak, cut across the grain into ¼- to ½-in. strips

1 TB. peanut oil

1 tsp. garlic powder

1 TB. fresh ginger, minced

2 TB. firmly packed brown sugar

1 TB. curry powder

¾ cup low-sodium fat-free beef broth

2 TB. reduced-sodium tamari or soy sauce

2 cups broccoli florets, cut into bite-size pieces

2 TB. dry-roasted peanuts, chopped

1. In a large, nonstick skillet over medium-high heat, combine flank steak and peanut oil. Cook, stirring often, for 6 to 8 minutes or until steak is browned.

2. Stir in garlic powder, ginger, brown sugar, curry powder, beef broth, and tamari. Reduce heat to medium-low. Toss in broccoli florets, cover, and cook, stirring occasionally, for 4 or 5 minutes.

3. Remove from heat, and garnish with chopped peanuts. Serve with your favorite rice dish.

Gut Facts

Ginger has been used in Asian cultures for thousands of years as a therapeutic herbal remedy to aid digestion, calm stomach upset, and minimize nausea and diarrhea. A cup of hot water simmered with a bit of peeled fresh ginger is a great antinausea remedy.

Beef Stir-Fry

This vibrant dish is so sweet and savory, you almost forget it's packed with good nutrition.

1 lb. flank steak, cut into thin strips across the grain

2 TB. peanut or vegetable oil

3 TB. reduced-sodium tamari or soy sauce

1 tsp. sesame oil

1 tsp. minced ginger

½ tsp. coriander

1 TB. brown sugar, firmly packed

1 cup snow peas, ends trimmed

2 medium carrots, peeled and cut into thin rounds

1 cup broccoli florets, cut into bite-size pieces

1 (8-oz.) can water chestnuts, sliced and drained

2 cups bean sprouts

Yield: 4 servings
Prep time: 15 minutes
Cook time: 11 to 13 minutes
Serving size: 2 cups
Each serving has:
400 calories
19.4 g carbohydrates
20 g fat
4 g fiber
35 g protein

1. In a large, nonstick skillet over medium heat, combine flank steak and peanut oil. Cook, stirring often, for 6 to 8 minutes or until steak is browned.

2. Stir in tamari, sesame oil, ginger, coriander, and brown sugar. Reduce heat to low, and simmer for 2 minutes.

3. Add snow peas, carrots, broccoli, water chestnuts, and bean sprouts. Cover and cook, stirring occasionally, for 3 more minutes. Enjoy served over brown or jasmine rice.

Gut Facts

Water chestnuts give a nice crunch to this dish. Nutritionally speaking, they're a good source of fiber and potassium.

Muchas Gracias Beef

This beef is packed with the flavors of Mexico, so plug in your slow cooker and treat your family to this spicy dish.

Yield: 8 servings
Prep time: 15 to 20 minutes
Cook time: 6 to 8 hours
Serving size: ¼ to 1 cup meat mixture
Each serving has:
271 calories
2 g carbohydrates
11.6 g fat
1 g fiber
38 g protein

1, 2 lb. pot roast, or brisket, trimmed of visible fat

1 TB. chili powder

2 tsp. cumin

1 tsp. onion salt

2 TB. olive or vegetable oil

1 (14.5-oz.) can diced tomatoes with green chilies

1 (14.5-oz.) can low-sodium fat-free beef broth

1. Place pot roast on a plate.

2. In a small bowl, combine chili powder, cumin, and onion salt. Rub spice mixture evenly over pot roast.

3. In a large stockpot over medium heat, add olive oil. Add pot roast, and cook, searing each side of meat to give it a good brown color, for about 3 or 4 minutes per side. Remove from heat.

4. Add tomatoes and beef broth to a slow cooker. Set temperature to low, add pot roast, cover, and cook for 6 to 8 hours.

5. Turn off slow cooker. Using two forks, shred meat inside the slow cooker, allowing it to mix with tomatoes and broth.

6. Enjoy meat over brown rice, or use a slotted spoon to remove meat and use as a filling in taco shells garnished with chopped tomatoes, lettuce, and grated reduced-fat cheddar cheese.

Gut Facts

Pot roasts don't fare well with dry cooking methods such as baking or roasting. To ensure a tender, moist meat, slow cook pot roast in liquid. Typical cuts for pot roast are brisket or rump roast.

Irish Shepherd's Pie

Lots of subtle flavors make this comfort food a family favorite. (My husband says he'd eat this every night of the week!)

6 medium red-skinned potatoes, peeled and quartered

¼ to ½ cup reduced-lactose low-fat milk

1 TB. butter or trans-fat-free margarine

2 TB. olive or vegetable oil

½ tsp. garlic salt

¼ tsp. freshly ground black pepper

½ tsp. onion salt

1 lb. extra-lean ground beef

1 large celery stalk, diced

2 medium carrots, peeled and sliced into thin rounds

½ tsp. ground thyme

2 TB. all-purpose flour

1 cup low-sodium fat-free beef broth

1 cup fresh or frozen peas, defrosted if frozen

2 TB. chopped fresh parsley

½ cup grated Irish cheddar (optional)

Yield: 6 servings
Prep time: 40 minutes
Cook time: 30 minutes
Serving size: ⅙ pie
Each serving has:
338 calories
35 g carbohydrates
13 g fat
4.5 g fiber
20 g protein

1. Preheat the oven to 350°F.

2. In a large stockpot, add potatoes, and fill the pot ¾ full of water. Set over high heat, and bring water to a boil. Boil potatoes for 15 to 20 minutes or until they're fork-tender.

3. Remove pot from heat, drain off water, and return the pot to the stove. Reduce heat to low.

4. Add ¼ to ½ cup milk, butter, 1 tablespoon olive oil, and garlic salt. Using a potato masher, mash potatoes for 2 or 3 minutes or until they're creamy. Use more or less milk to reach desired creamy consistency.

5. In a large, nonstick skillet over medium heat, add ground beef, celery, carrots, remaining 1 tablespoon olive oil, and thyme. Cook, stirring frequently to chop meat and ensure even cooking, for 8 to 10 minutes. Remove from heat and drain excess fat.

6. Return the skillet to the stove, and increase heat to medium. Sprinkle meat with flour, and slowly pour in beef broth. Increase heat to medium-high, and cook, stirring, for 2 or 3 minutes to make gravy. Add peas and parsley, cook for 1 more minute, and remove from heat.

7. Place meat mixture in a 9-inch pie plate, and cover evenly with mashed potatoes. Bake for 20 minutes. Remove from the oven, and top with grated cheese (if using). Return to the stove, and cook for 10 more minutes. If not using cheese, bake uninterrupted for 30 minutes.

8. Let sit for 5 to 10 minutes, cut into 6 wedges, and enjoy with a colorful salad.

Variation: If you can't find Irish cheddar, you can use regular cheddar instead.

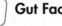 **Gut Facts**

Traditionally made mashed potatoes are a source of lactose, thanks to the milk. I've modified this recipe to minimize any troublesome lactose. Cheddar cheese has little to no lactose, so it shouldn't pose any problem for the lactose intolerant.

17

Pork and Poultry

In This Chapter

- ◆ Palate-pleasing pork
- ◆ Protein-packed dishes
- ◆ Outside-the-box chicken recipes
- ◆ Lean and tasty poultry dishes

This is the white meat chapter. Known for their lower fat content, pork and poultry often live up to their reputation. But buyers beware: not all cuts of "white meat" are lean. And depending on how you choose to cook it, these meats could easily go from lean and mean to fried and fatty!

In this chapter, you'll find loads of recipes incorporating lean cuts of pork and poultry in tempting and still low-fat ways. I've even included a few traditional favorites, modified so they're a bit easier on your digestive tract!

Pork, Pork, Pork

Lean cuts of pork are low-fat and tasty meal options. From a nutritional standpoint, pork packs a mighty punch as a great source of protein, iron, niacin, riboflavin, and vitamins B_6 and B_{12}. So scope out pork at your favorite grocery store, and be sure to choose lean cuts of pork such as tenderloin, center-cut chops, top loin, center loin, Canadian bacon, and 90- to 95-percent-lean boneless ham.

Pork's naturally light flavor makes it a wonderful complement to both sweet and savory ingredients. In this chapter, you'll find so many different ways to enjoy lean and healthy pork dishes.

Popular Poultry

Chicken is such a versatile protein source. Naturally tender, it requires very little preparation prior to cooking. Take a peek at the many fabulous chicken entrée recipes in this chapter. I bet you'll never tire of this delicious—and versatile—lean meat.

Digestibles _____

A little fat goes a long way for taste and flavor; just don't go overboard. Simple tricks such as trimming visible fat and skin away from meats helps reduce your fat intake. If you must cook with the skin on, season meat under the skin for added taste—and less temptation to eat the flavored skin.

Great picks for chicken include, of course, boneless, skinless breast for its ease of preparation and very low fat content. Thigh meat has a bit more fat but offers a different flavor and is available skinless for a nice alternative.

Consider swapping out your ground beef and opt for ground chicken or ground turkey breast. You won't be sorry, and you'll save a few fat grams along the way.

And don't be fooled into thinking roasted turkey is just for the holidays. You can enjoy this tasty meat any time of the year! For a wonderful quicker-fix alternative to roasting a whole bird, try turkey tenderloin, which cooks up in a snap!

Grilled Pork Tenderloin

Seasoned to perfection, a hint of sweet, and a nice blend of spice make this tenderloin absolutely mouthwatering.

1 (2-lb.) pork tenderloin, or 2 (1-lb.) tenderloins

2 TB. Dijon mustard

2 tsp. finely chopped fresh thyme

1 tsp. garlic salt

1 tsp. onion powder

1 tsp. brown sugar, firmly packed

1 tsp. paprika

½ tsp. freshly ground black pepper

1 TB. olive or vegetable oil

1. Evenly coat outside of pork with Dijon mustard. Set aside.

2. In a small bowl, combine thyme, garlic salt, onion powder, brown sugar, paprika, and pepper, and blend with fork. Rub spice mixture all over pork, pressing in and coating evenly.

3. Drizzle pork with olive oil to lightly coat. Let sit for 10 to 20 minutes.

4. Preheat the grill.

5. Place pork on the grill over medium-low heat, and cook for 20 to 30 minutes, flipping about every 5 minutes, or until an instant-read thermometer inserted into the center registers 160°F.

6. Remove pork from the grill, cover with aluminum foil, and let sit for 10 minutes. Slice into 24 slices. Consider serving with Smashed Potatoes and Peppers and Mushroom Medley (both recipes in Chapter 19).

Yield: 8 servings

Prep time: 10 minutes plus 20 to 30 minutes rest time

Cook time: 30 minutes

Serving size: 3 slices

Each serving has:

143 calories

1 g carbohydrates

4 g fat

0 g fiber

24 g protein

Gut Facts

Dry rubs are a great way to flavor meat. Try concocting your own mixture with your favorite herbs and seasoning.

Center-Cut Dijon Pork Chops

You'll love this wonderful way to serve chops—moist, mustardy, and scrumptious!

Yield: 4 chops
Prep time: 5 minutes
Cook time: 25 to 30 minutes
Serving size: 1 chop
Each serving has:
350 calories
10 g carbohydrates
17 g fat
1 g fiber
37 g protein

4 (½-in.-thick) center-cut pork chops

2 TB. Dijon mustard

½ cup Italian-style bread-crumbs

1 TB. butter or trans-fat-free margarine, melted

1 TB. olive oil

1. Preheat the oven to 350°F. Spray a cookie sheet with nonstick cooking spray.

2. Arrange pork chops on the prepared cookie sheet, and spread about ½ tablespoon Dijon mustard on each chop.

3. In a small bowl, combine breadcrumbs with melted butter and olive oil. Evenly distribute crumbs on top of pork chops.

4. Bake for 25 to 30 minutes or until chops are cooked through and no longer pink. Enjoy with Sweet Potato Fries (recipe in Chapter 19) and Bibb Lettuce Salad with Dijon Vinaigrette (recipe in Chapter 14).

Gut Facts

Center-cut chops are a lean and low-fat cut of pork. And they cook quickly, so they're perfect for busy weeknight meals.

Pork Chop Simmer with Tri-Colored Peppers

Colorful peppers add a fruity and tangy combo to this dish.

4 (½-in.-thick) center-cut boneless chops

½ cup all-purpose flour

½ tsp. freshly ground black pepper

½ tsp. onion salt

2 TB. olive or vegetable oil

1 medium red bell pepper, ribs and seeds removed, and cut into strips

1 medium yellow bell pepper, ribs and seeds removed, and cut into strips

1 medium green bell pepper, ribs and seeds removed, and cut into strips

Yield: 4 servings
Prep time: 10 minutes
Cook time: 22 to 25 minutes
Serving size: 1 pork chop
Each serving has:
379 calories
17 g carbohydrates
17 g fat
2.4 g fiber
37 g protein

1. In a large zipper-lock bag, combine 1 chop, flour, pepper, and onion salt. Close the bag, and give it a good shake to coat chop. Shaking off any excess flour, remove chop to a plate. Continue with remaining 3 chops. Discard any extra flour and pepper mixture.

2. In a large, nonstick skillet over medium heat, combine 1 tablespoon olive oil, red bell pepper, yellow bell pepper, and green bell pepper. Cook for 5 to 8 minutes or until wilted. Remove peppers to clean plate.

3. Add pork chops and remaining 1 tablespoon olive oil to the skillet, set over medium heat, and cook chops for 5 minutes per side.

4. Add peppers back to skillet to warm for about 2 or 3 minutes, and serve immediately. These chops are terrific with a side of Sweet Potato Fries and Stuffed Tomatoes (recipes in Chapter 19).

Tummy Trouble

Bell peppers are one of the Environmental Working Group's "dirty dozen" of foods that have the most pesticide residues. Also on the list, starting with the worst offenders: peaches, apples, celery, nectarines, strawberries, cherries, kale, lettuce, grapes (imported), carrots, and pears. To decrease pesticide intake, always wash produce and consider purchasing the organic versions of these foods.

Pork Carnitas

This is a terrific Mexican dish with caramelized meat in every sweet and spicy mouthful.

Yield: 8 servings
Prep time: 5 minutes
Cook time: 60 to 62 minutes
Serving size: 4 slices
Each serving has:
455 calories
24 g carbohydrates
29 g fat
3 g fiber
22 g protein

2 lb. boneless pork roast, trimmed of visible fat and cut into 1-in. pieces

2 TB. olive or vegetable oil

1 tsp. garlic salt

1 (14.5-oz.) can reduced-sodium fat-free beef broth

6 cups water

$\frac{1}{4}$ cup dry red wine

$\frac{1}{2}$ cup orange juice

$\frac{1}{2}$ cup reduced-lactose low-fat milk

1 tsp. chili powder

$\frac{1}{2}$ tsp. ground cumin

16 (6-in.) corn tortillas, warmed

Gut Facts

A Mexican-style dish, *carnitas* means "little pieces of meat."

1. In a large stockpot over medium heat, combine pork, olive oil, and garlic salt. Cook for about 10 minutes to brown pork.

2. Slowly add beef broth and water, and bring to a boil. Reduce heat to low, cover, and simmer for 40 minutes. Drain any residual broth and water.

3. Return the pot to medium heat, and add red wine, orange juice, milk, chili powder, and cumin. Cook for 10 to 12 minutes or until all liquid is evaporated.

4. Slice meat into about 32 slices, and serve meat inside warmed tortillas.

Marinated Pork Roast

You'll love the aromatic pleasures this pork roast provides. This dish requires overnight marinating, but it's worth it!

4 lb. pork shoulder, trimmed of visible fat

½ cup reduced-sodium tamari or soy sauce

½ cup red wine

2 cloves garlic, cut in half

1 TB. dry mustard

1 tsp. ground ginger

1 tsp. ground thyme

Yield: 16 servings
Prep time: 10 minutes plus overnight marinate time
Cook time: 2 to 2½ hours
Serving size: 2 slices
Each serving has:
316 calories
1 g carbohydrates
24 g fat
0 g fiber
24 g protein

1. In an extra-large zipper-lock bag or glass bowl, combine pork roast, tamari, red wine, garlic, dry mustard, ginger, and thyme. Close the bag, and give it a good shake to mix. Place the bag in the refrigerator to marinate overnight.

2. Preheat the oven to 325°F.

3. Remove pork from the bag. Save marinade and return to the refrigerator. Remove and discard garlic pieces.

4. Place roast in a 9×13 pan, and cook, uncovered, for 1½ hours.

5. Remove from the oven, and drizzle leftover marinade over pork. Cook for another ½ to 1 hour or until an instant-read thermometer inserted into the center reads 160°F.

6. Slice roast into about 32 slices, and enjoy with baked potatoes and Yellow Summer Squash with Bacon (recipe in Chapter 19).

Digestibles

Be sure to trim the roast of all visible fat. This lowers the fat content tremendously. The pork shoulder works nicely in this recipe but does have a bit more fat than pork tenderloin.

Chelsea's Favorite Slow Cooker BBQ Pork

Tomatoes and spice infuse this sweet and tasty pulled pork.

Yield: 4 servings
Prep time: 10 minutes
Cook time: 4 hours
Serving size: ¼ mixture
Each serving has:
385 calories
39 g carbohydrates
9.5 g fat
0 g fiber
34.5 g protein

1 lb. center-cut pork chops, cut into bite-size chunks

1 (12-oz.) jar barbecue sauce

1. In a slow cooker, combine pork and barbecue sauce. Set the temperature to low, and slow cook for 4 hours.

2. Shred meat by using 2 forks to pull meat apart. Serve as filling for sandwiches on crusty rolls or alongside brown rice and your favorite vegetable dish.

Digestibles

Choose a slow cooker recipe when you have limited time for meal preparation. There's something to be said for coming home to a hot cooked meal ready to eat. I like this pork with the microwavable brown rice that's ready in just 3 or 4 minutes. And when you're shopping for barbecue sauce, look for one made without high-fructose corn syrup.

Pork Medallions and Savory Sauce

This simple, tender meat comes with a delectable sauce as a bonus.

1 lb. pork tenderloin, cut into about 24 ($\frac{1}{2}$-in.) rounds

$\frac{1}{2}$ tsp. onion salt

$\frac{1}{2}$ tsp. freshly ground black pepper

2 TB. olive or vegetable oil

1 to 1$\frac{1}{2}$ cups low-sodium fat-free chicken broth

2 TB. *Dijon mustard*

1 TB. cornstarch

2 TB. chopped fresh parsley

Yield: 4 servings
Prep time: 10 minutes
Cook time: 10 to 12 minutes
Serving size: 6 rounds
Each serving has:
198 calories
2 g carbohydrates
11 g fat
0 g fiber
24 g protein

1. Sprinkle pork with onion salt and pepper.

2. In a large, nonstick skillet over medium heat, add olive oil. Add pork in an even layer, and cook for 3 or 4 minutes per side or until an instant-read thermometer inserted into the center reads 160°F. Transfer pork to a plate.

3. In the skillet, mix 1 cup chicken broth and Dijon mustard with a fork. Increase heat to medium-high, and slowly incorporate cornstarch, stirring constantly, for about 2 minutes or until mixture is thickened to the consistency of gravy, adding more broth as necessary.

4. Reduce heat to low, return pork to the skillet, and cook for 2 more minutes. Garnish with parsley, and serve.

Wellness Words

Dijon mustard was first made in Dijon, France. This light yellow mustard has a stronger flavor compared with most American mustards.

Chicken Piccata

My guests love this lovely, light lemon- and wine-infused chicken.

Yield: *4 servings*
Prep time: 15 minutes
Cook time: 20 minutes
Serving size: 2 cutlets
Each serving has:
405 calories
29 g carbohydrates
18 g fat
.8 g fiber
27 g protein

Digestibles

Chicken or veal can be used in this piccata recipe, which is traditionally made with a wine and lemon sauce.

1 cup all-purpose flour

½ tsp. onion salt

½ tsp. freshly ground black pepper

8 boneless, skinless chicken breast cutlets (about 1 lb.)

3 TB. olive or vegetable oil

2 TB. butter

1 (14.5-oz.) can low-sodium fat-free chicken broth

⅓ cup freshly squeezed lemon juice (2 lemons)

2 TB. brined capers

¼ cup white wine (optional)

2 TB. cornstarch

⅓ cup chopped fresh parsley

1. In a large zipper-lock bag, combine flour, onion salt, pepper, and 1 chicken breast. Close the bag, and give it a good shake to coat chicken. Shaking off any excess flour, remove chicken to wax paper. Do not overlap chicken or it will stick together. Continue with remaining chicken. Discard any leftover flour mixture.

2. In a large skillet over medium heat, combine 2 tablespoons olive oil and 1 tablespoon butter. When the pan is hot and butter has melted, add a layer of chicken cutlets. Cook for about 5 minutes, turn chicken over, and cook for 2 or 3 more minutes. Remove cooked chicken to a plate, and continue with remaining chicken, adding remaining 1 tablespoon olive oil and 1 tablespoon butter as needed.

3. Increase heat to medium-high, and stir in chicken broth, lemon juice, capers, and white wine. Slowly whisk in cornstarch to blend and thicken sauce.

4. Add chicken back to the pan, and gently coat pieces with lemon-wine sauce. Garnish with parsley, and enjoy with a side of your favorite pasta and garden salad.

Chicken Saltimbocca

This light and tangy Italian chicken dish includes an added bonus of prosciutto.

1 cup all-purpose flour

1 tsp. garlic salt

½ tsp. freshly ground black pepper

8 boneless, skinless chicken breast cutlets (about 1 lb.)

3 TB. olive oil

2 TB. butter

1 (14.5-oz.) can low-sodium fat-free chicken broth

⅓ cup freshly squeezed lemon juice (1 or 2 lemons)

2 cups button mushrooms, sliced

½ cup white wine

1 TB. cornstarch

4 thinly sliced pieces prosciutto

2 TB. finely chopped fresh parsley

Yield: 4 servings	
Prep time: 15 minutes	
Cook time: 20 minutes	
Serving size: 2 cutlets	
Each serving has:	
435 calories	
30 g carbohydrates	
19 g fat	
1.3 g fiber	
31 g protein	

Gut Facts

Saltimbocca means "jumps in mouth" in Italian, probably because you want it to jump into your mouth because it tastes so good! This popular Italian dish can be made with veal, chicken, or shrimp.

1. In a large zipper-lock bag, combine flour, garlic salt, pepper, and 1 chicken breast. Close the bag, and give it a good shake to coat chicken. Shaking off any excess flour, remove chicken to wax paper. Do not overlap chicken or it will stick together. Continue with remaining chicken. Discard any leftover flour mixture.

2. In a large skillet over medium heat, combine 2 tablespoons olive oil and 1 tablespoon butter. When the pan is hot and butter has melted, add a layer of chicken cutlets. Cook for about 5 minutes, turn chicken over, and cook for 2 or 3 more minutes. Remove cooked chicken to a plate, and continue with remaining chicken, adding remaining 1 tablespoon olive oil and 1 tablespoon butter as needed.

3. In another large skillet over medium heat, combine chicken broth, lemon juice, and mushrooms. Stir and cook for about 5 minutes.

4. In a small bowl, whisk together white wine and cornstarch. Add to mushrooms, and increase heat to medium-high. Cook, whisking constantly, for 3 to 5 minutes.

5. Add chicken back to the pan, and top with prosciutto. Garnish with parsley, and enjoy with a side of pasta or rice.

Grilled Chicken Kabobs

Light the grill! These grilled chicken kabobs feature the best veggies from the garden and are a cookout favorite.

Yield: 8 skewers
Prep time: 15 minutes plus 4 hours marinate time
Cook time: 8 to 10 minutes
Serving size: 2 skewers
Each serving has:
237 calories
11 g carbohydrates
9 g fat
3.3 g fiber
28 g protein

1 lb. boneless, skinless chicken breast, cut into bite-size chunks

¼ cup olive or vegetable oil

4 TB. freshly squeezed lemon juice (1 lemon)

1 TB. chopped fresh thyme

1 tsp. garlic salt

½ tsp. freshly ground black pepper

1 medium zucchini, skin on, cut into ½-in. circles and then cut in half

8 bamboo skewers, soaked in water

1½ cups cherry tomatoes

1 large green bell pepper, ribs and seeds removed, and cut into bite-size chunks

3 cups white button mushrooms, ends trimmed (16 mushrooms)

Gut Facts

Did you know: marinating with acidic ingredients such as lemon juice, tomatoes, wine, and vinegars is a great way to infuse flavor while tenderizing meat.

1. In a large zipper-lock bag, combine chicken, olive oil, lemon juice, thyme, garlic salt, pepper, and zucchini. Close the bag, and give it a good shake to coat chicken. Place the bag in the refrigerator for 4 hours to marinate.

2. Preheat the grill.

3. Thread the skewers in the following order: chicken, cherry tomato, bell pepper, chicken, zucchini, and mushroom. Repeat another sequence on same skewer and then start a new skewer.

4. Grill skewers for 5 minutes, turn, and cook 5 more minutes. To ensure safe cooking, be sure chicken is no longer pink and an instant-read thermometer inserted into the center reads 165°F.

Asian Chicken Lettuce Wraps

Lettuce serves as a little serving dish for this fragrant and flavorful Asian-infused chicken.

1 medium head iceberg lettuce

2 TB. sesame oil

1 TB. olive oil

1½ lb. ground chicken breast

2 TB. cornstarch

2 TB. freshly grated ginger

1 tsp. garlic powder

1 medium stalk *lemongrass*, finely chopped

2 TB. reduced-sodium tamari or soy sauce

1 small head bok choy, ribs and leaves finely sliced

2 TB. finely chopped fresh cilantro

Yield: 6 servings
Prep time: 15 minutes
Cook time: 15 minutes
Serving size: 1 cup meat mixture and 3 or 4 lettuce leaves
Each serving has:
239 calories
4 g carbohydrates
15 g fat
trace fiber
20 g protein

1. Cut lettuce in half, and discard outer leaves. Wash thoroughly, wrap in a clean dish towel, and place in the refrigerator to keep cold and crisp.

2. In a large, nonstick skillet over medium heat, combine sesame oil and olive oil. Add chicken, and immediately sprinkle with cornstarch. Cook, stirring, for 3 to 5 minutes.

3. Add ginger, garlic powder, lemongrass, soy sauce, and bok choy. Reduce heat to low, and stir to combine all ingredients. Simmer for 1 minute to wilt bok choy, and garnish with fresh cilantro.

4. Place lettuce on the table and serve with chicken mixture on the side. Scoop mixture into lettuce, wrap, and enjoy with a side of brown rice.

 Wellness Words _____

Lemongrass, a long, yellow stalk, is a tropical grass commonly used in Asian dishes, and adds a delightful lemon flavor to this dish. You can substitute 1 teaspoon grated lemon rind for the lemongrass if necessary. Asian markets or health food stores are most likely to stock lemongrass.

Curried Chicken Salad

This sweet and spicy chicken makes wonderful salad or sandwich filler.

Yield: 6 servings
Prep time: 10 minutes
Serving size: ¾ cup
Each serving has:
211 calories
5 g carbohydrates
11.7 g fat
.6 g fiber
21 g protein

3 cups cooked chicken breast, cut into bite-size chunks

½ cup light mayonnaise

1 cup red grapes, cut in half

¼ cup pecans, chopped

1 tsp. curry powder

½ tsp. onion salt

1. In a medium bowl, gently combine chicken, mayonnaise, red grapes, pecans, curry powder, and onion salt.

2. Refrigerate chicken salad for 1 hour. Enjoy over salad greens or in a sandwich.

Gut Facts

Red grapes are a source of resveratrol, a powerful antioxidant that's been shown in studies to possibly lower risk of obesity and diabetes. Some research suggests resveratrol may have anti-inflammatory effects as well.

Chicken Chop Suey

My son Brennan loves this dish. Lots of vegetables make it a low-calorie dish with lots of flavor.

1 lb. boneless, skinless chicken breast, cut into bite-size chunks

2 TB. peanut or vegetable oil

4 medium carrots, peeled and sliced into thin rounds

¼ cup water

2 TB. cornstarch

5 TB. reduced-sodium tamari or soy sauce

5 medium stalks celery, sliced

2 cups white button mushrooms, sliced

2 cups bean sprouts

Yield: 4 servings
Prep time: 15 minutes
Cook time: 14 to 16 minutes
Serving size: 2 cups
Each serving has:
268 calories
17 g carbohydrates
9 g fat
4.2 g fiber
28 g protein

1. In a large skillet over medium heat, combine chicken and peanut oil. Cook, stirring, for 8 to 10 minutes or until chicken is no longer pink.

2. Reduce heat to low. Add carrots, and slowly pour in water. Cover, and cook, stirring occasionally, for 2 minutes.

3. In a small bowl, whisk together cornstarch and soy sauce. Pour soy sauce over chicken and carrots, increase heat to medium, and stir for 1 minute.

4. Mix in celery, mushrooms, and bean sprouts. Reduce heat to low, and cook, covered and stirring occasionally, for 2 or 3 more minutes. Enjoy with brown rice.

Gut Facts _____

A bit more pricey than vegetable oil, peanut oil is rich in monounsaturated fats, and therefore considered a heart-healthy fat. Peanut oil adds a nutty flavor to this dish.

Chicken Satay with Peanut Dipping Sauce

Serve this versatile dish as appetizers for a crowd or a fun evening meal. The flavors of Thailand infuse the meat and dipping sauce.

Yield: 4 servings
Prep time: 10 to 15 minutes plus overnight marinate time
Cook time: 10 minutes
Serving size: 4 or 5 skewers plus ¼ cup peanut sauce
Each serving has:
479 calories
21 g carbohydrates
30 g fat
1.2 g fiber
34 g protein

Gut Facts

Satay is a popular southeast Asian dish made of marinated meat served on skewers.

1 lb. boneless, skinless chicken breast, cut into about 20 thin strips big enough to thread on a skewer

½ cup plus 1 TB. reduced-sodium tamari

⅓ cup sesame oil

¼ cup dark brown sugar, firmly packed

3 TB. freshly squeezed lemon juice (2 lemons)

1 tsp. garlic powder

1 TB. coriander

20 bamboo skewers, soaked in water

⅓ cup creamy peanut butter

1 cup reduced-sodium fat-free chicken broth

1½ tsp. light brown sugar, packed

½ tsp. ground ginger

¼ tsp. crushed red pepper flakes

1. In a large zipper-lock bag, combine chicken, ½ cup tamari, sesame oil, dark brown sugar, 2 tablespoons lemon juice, garlic powder, and coriander. Close the bag, and give it a good shake to blend. Place the bag in the refrigerator to marinate overnight.

2. Preheat the grill.

3. Thread chicken on skewers, weaving meat in and out. Grill for 3 to 5 minutes per side or until cooked through. Place cooked skewers on a large, clean plate and cover with aluminum foil to keep warm.

4. In a small saucepan over medium heat, combine peanut butter, chicken broth, remaining 1 tablespoon lemon juice, brown sugar, remaining 1 tablespoon tamari, ginger, and crushed pepper. Cook, stirring for about 2 minutes. Serve sauce alongside skewers.

Parmesan-Crusted Chicken

Crispy and cheesy, this quick-fix chicken is a family favorite!

4 boneless, skinless chicken breasts (about 1 lb.)

3 cups cornflake cereal

1 cup grated Parmesan cheese

$\frac{1}{2}$ **tsp. onion salt**

1 TB. dried parsley

1 large egg

$\frac{1}{2}$ **cup water**

Yield: 4 servings
Prep time: 10 minutes
Cook time: 20 to 25 minutes
Serving size: 1 breast
Each serving has:
322 calories
19 g carbohydrates
10 g fat
.5 g fiber
36 g protein

1. Preheat the oven to 350°F. Spray a nonstick cookie sheet with nonstick cooking spray.

2. In a large zipper-lock bag, combine cornflakes, Parmesan cheese, onion salt, and parsley. Close the bag, being sure not to fill it with too much air. Using your hands, crunch cereal inside the bag until cornflakes are crumbled and ingredients are mixed.

3. In a small, shallow bowl, whisk together egg and water. Dip chicken individually into egg mixture and then into the bag with cornflake crumbs. Press chicken into crumbs to create a crust. Place chicken on the prepared cookie sheet.

4. Bake for 20 to 25 minutes or until cooked through. Enjoy this crispy chicken with mashed potatoes and Steamed Broccoli with Sesame Dressing (recipe in Chapter 19).

Digestibles

The crunchy cereal gives this chicken a nice, crispy exterior. For another alternative, swap 1 $\frac{1}{2}$ cups breadcrumbs for the cornflake cereal.

Ground Chicken Taco Lasagna

There's no need to boil any water for "pasta" in this lasagna recipe. This quick-fix meal is loaded with tasty Mexican flavors, chili powder for a kick, and a bit of smoky essence from the cumin.

Yield: 6 servings	
Prep time: 10 minutes	
Cook time: 15 minutes	
Serving size: ⅙ pan	
Each serving has:	
303 calories	
18 g carbohydrates	
16 g fat	
2.8 g fiber	
22 g protein	

Gut Facts

This recipe is adapted from Kathleen Daeleman's recipe for Chicken Taco Casserole in her book *Getting Thin and Loving Food!* Her cookbook is one of my favorites.

1 lb. ground chicken breast	¼ tsp. freshly ground black pepper
1 (14.5-oz.) can diced tomatoes	8 (6-in.) corn tortillas
1 TB. chili powder	1½ cups finely grated cheddar cheese
1 tsp. ground cumin	2 cups shredded iceberg lettuce
½ tsp. onion salt	

1. Preheat the oven to 350°F.

2. In a large, nonstick skillet over medium heat, add ground chicken and chop with the end of a spatula into small, crumb-size bits. Cook for 2 or 3 minutes or until chicken is mostly white and cooked through.

3. Open the can of tomatoes, drain juice into the bottom of a 9×13 pan, and add drained tomatoes to the skillet. Add chili powder, cumin, onion salt, and pepper to the skillet, stirring to blend. Reduce heat to low, and simmer for 2 minutes, stirring occasionally.

4. In the 9×13 pan with tomato juice, layer 4 tortillas, somewhat overlapping. Add ½ of meat mixture, and top with ½ cup cheese. Layer 4 more tortillas on top of cheese, layer with remaining meat, top with an even layer of remaining cheese. Cover with aluminum foil.

5. Bake for 15 minutes or until cheese is fully melted. Garnish with shredded lettuce, cut into 6 even pieces, and enjoy!

Ground Turkey Meatloaf

Let's talk comfort food! This version of traditional meatloaf offers a tasty, low-fat alternative.

2 lb. ground turkey breast

1 cup wheat or gluten-free breadcrumbs

½ cup grated Parmesan cheese

2 large eggs, beaten

1 medium red bell pepper, ribs and seeds removed, and finely chopped

2 tsp. Italian seasoning

1 tsp. onion salt

Yield: 8 servings
Prep time: 10 minutes
Cook time: 50 to 60 minutes
Serving size: ⅛ pan
Each serving has:
223 calories
11 g carbohydrates
5 g fat
1 g fiber
33 g protein

1. Preheat the oven to 350°F. Spray a 9×5×3-inch loaf pan with nonstick cooking spray.

2. In a large mixing bowl, combine ground turkey, breadcrumbs, Parmesan cheese, eggs, red bell pepper, Italian seasoning, and onion salt. Mix well with spoon. Place meat mixture in the prepared loaf pan, pressing down to fill the pan evenly.

3. Bake for 50 to 60 minutes or until an instant-read thermometer inserted into the center reads 165°F. Cut into 8 even pieces. Enjoy with Smashed Potatoes (recipe in Chapter 19) and a green salad for a nice comfort meal.

 Digestibles _____

If you don't think your family will go for a full-turkey version meatloaf, try mixing 1 pound ground turkey breast with 1 pound 90-percent-extra-lean hamburger in this recipe. No one will notice you added the ground turkey!

Turkey Tenderloin

The spicy and creamy marinade keeps the turkey moist and delicious, even when prepared on the grill.

Yield: 6 servings
Prep time: 5 minutes plus 4 to 6 hours or overnight marinate time
Cook time: 26 minutes
Serving size: about 4 rounds
Each serving has:
125 calories
2 g carbohydrates
1 g fat
0 g fiber
25.5 g protein

¾ cup plain nonfat Greek yogurt

2 tsp. chili powder

1 tsp. cumin

1 tsp. coriander

1 tsp. onion salt

¼ tsp. paprika

1 TB. freshly squeezed lime juice (1 lime)

1½ lb. turkey tenderloin

1. In a small bowl, combine yogurt, chili powder, cumin, coriander, onion salt, paprika, and lime juice.

2. In a large zipper-lock bag, combine turkey and yogurt mixture. Close the bag, and give it a good shake to disperse marinade. Place the bag in the refrigerator to marinate for 4 to 6 hours or overnight.

3. Preheat the grill.

4. Remove turkey from the bag, discard marinade, wrap turkey in aluminum foil, and grill for 8 minutes. Flip over turkey, and grill for 8 more minutes. Carefully remove the aluminum foil, and grill for 5 more minutes per side or until turkey is no longer pink and an instant-read thermometer inserted into the center reads 165°F.

5. Slice into 24 thin rounds, and serve with Ann's Cumin Corn with Cilantro (recipe in Chapter 19) and possibly some fragrant basmati rice.

Gut Facts

Yogurt marinades are popular in Indian cooking and are known as *tandoori*. This yogurt-and-citrus marinade works as a meat tenderizer and keeps the meat moist while it cooks.

Chapter **18**

Perfect Pasta and Pizza

In This Chapter

- ◆ Plan on pasta
- ◆ Wow them with wheat-free pasta
- ◆ Impressive pizzas with pizzazz
- ◆ The secret to easy pizza-making

I'm married to an Italian, so I often joke to my friends that my marriage came packaged with a bottle of olive oil. Maybe a bit of pasta and pizza thrown in, too, if I have to be completely honest! Pasta and pizza are notably heavy-handed in the starch and carbohydrate category, so to balance out your meal, be sure to also include colorful veggies and lean protein choices.

In this chapter, I give you a flurry of vegetables introduced into your favorite pasta and pizza meals. In addition to all the vitamins and minerals they provide, their fiber boost will keep your belly fuller longer and likely keep your intestines a bit more regular. I promise you and your family will love these healthier versions of pizza and pasta meals.

Pasta Dishes Even Italians Will Envy!

With its easy preparation, pasta makes meal-planning in a pinch quite simple. As a rich source of carbohydrates, pasta provides your body with energy, so don't be afraid to add a few more noodles in your life! Try whole-grain wheat pasta, if you tolerate wheat, for an extra fiber kick. For those with wheat intolerance, try substituting corn or rice pasta for all your favorite pasta meals.

It's easy to overindulge on pasta, so don't rush to cook more pasta than you need. Simply boil what you need, or if you make a big portion, store the extra servings in the refrigerator and away from temptation. A 1 or 1½ cup portion is generally ample for most adults.

Peace, Love, and Pizzas

Who doesn't love pizza? In addition to the taste, I love the ease of making pizza for a quick-fix meal. For years, I used to roll out the dough with a rolling pin and flour, creating a mess each and every time. The day I saw Emeril Lagasse reveal on TV his quicker version of pizza-making changed all of that!

To make pizza in a snap, start with a shallow bowl drizzled with about 1 table-spoon of oil, add the pizza dough, and let it sit for 5 minutes. Flip it over and allow the other side of the dough to get some oil coverage. Then, carry the dough over to your kitchen sink and stretch it out with your hands. (Working over the sink helps catch any oil that may drop off the dough.) Gently widen the dough into the shape of your pizza dish or jelly-roll pan, and voilà! No more rolling pin or flour, and far less mess!

There are no special rules when it comes to making pizza, so create what appeals to you. If wheat isn't your friend, try gluten-free pizza crusts. You can find gluten-free crusts in the freezer section of some grocery stores or at health food stores. Have fun, and be healthy!

Farmer's Market Pasta Salad

My friend Liz adds vibrant colored produce to all her favorite dishes. This beautiful veggie-full pasta salad is one of her inspirations.

1 lb. short or medium whole-wheat, white, corn, or rice pasta

1 (14.5-oz.) can kidney or black beans, rinsed and drained

¼ cup onion- and garlic-free Italian dressing

1 medium red bell pepper, ribs and seeds removed, and cut into bite-size chunks

1 medium yellow bell pepper, ribs and seeds removed, and cut into bite-size chunks

1 medium orange bell pepper, ribs and seeds removed, and cut into bite-size chunks

2 cups cherry or grape tomatoes, cut in half

4 cups fresh sugar snap peas, ends trimmed and cut in half

2 medium carrots, peeled and sliced into thin rounds

2 TB. finely chopped fresh parsley

Yield: 12 to 14 servings
Prep time: 20 minutes
Cook time: 8 to 15 minutes
Serving size: 1½ cups
Each serving has:
195 calories
37 g carbohydrates
2 g fat
5 g fiber
7.5 g protein

1. Cook pasta according to package directions. Drain, and rinse in warm water to keep warm.

2. In a large bowl, gently combine kidney beans, Italian dressing, red bell pepper, yellow bell pepper, orange bell pepper, tomatoes, sugar snap peas, and carrots.

3. Add warm pasta to vegetables, stir, and garnish with parsley. Serve warm, or refrigerate for an equally tasty cold pasta salad.

 Gut Facts

Despite their sweet taste, sugar snap peas are actually low in sugar. They add a wonderful crunch to this pasta salad and make a great snack on the go. Simply wash and trim ends, toss into a zipper-lock bag, and out the door you go.

Our Favorite Tomato-Basil Pasta

This tasty pasta dish is at its best when made with vine-ripened seasonal tomatoes. The recipe is inspired by my friend Pattie, who was born an American but is every bit Italian.

Yield: 6 servings
Prep time: 10 minutes
Cook time: 8 to 15 minutes
Serving size: 1 cup
Each serving has:
189 calories
31 g carbohydrates
5.5 g fat
2.3 g fiber
5 g protein

½ lb. whole-wheat, white, corn, or rice *penne* pasta

4 medium tomatoes, chopped into bite-size chunks

2 TB. olive or vegetable oil

1 tsp. garlic powder

½ tsp. onion salt

1 cup fresh basil, sliced into thin strips

1. Cook pasta according to package directions. Drain, rinse, and keep warm.

2. In a medium serving dish, combine tomatoes, olive oil, garlic powder, onion salt, and basil. Add warm pasta, and gently mix.

3. Let pasta sit on countertop for 30 minutes before serving. Refrigerate leftovers—this pasta salad is wonderful cold, too!

Wellness Words

Penne is short, tube-shape pasta with diagonal-cut ends. In Latin, *penne* means "feather" or "quill."

Alfredo Pasta with Shrimp and Spinach

Now you, too, can enjoy alfredo! Here, a creamy, cheesy-garlicy sauce pairs with pasta, spinach, and shrimp.

1 lb. whole-wheat, white, corn, or rice spaghetti or linguini pasta

1 lb. (16 to 20) extra-large shrimp, peeled and deveined

1 TB. butter

1 TB. olive or vegetable oil

2 TB. all-purpose flour

2 cups reduced-lactose low-fat milk

$\frac{1}{2}$ cup Parmesan cheese, grated

1 tsp. garlic powder

$\frac{1}{2}$ tsp. freshly ground black pepper

1 (10-oz.) pkg. frozen spinach, defrosted and squeezed of excess water

Yield: 8 servings
Prep time: 5 minutes
Cook time: 8 to 15 minutes
Serving size: $1\frac{1}{2}$ cups
Each serving has:
361 calories
48.5 g carbohydrates
8 g fat
3 g fiber
24 g protein

1. Cook pasta according to package directions. During the last 5 minutes of boiling time, add shrimp. Before draining pasta, remove 1 shrimp and cut in half to test for doneness. Thoroughly cooked shrimp are pink and opaque in the center. Drain and rinse pasta and shrimp and add to large serving bowl. Cover with aluminum foil to keep warm.

2. In a medium saucepan over medium heat, combine butter, olive oil, and flour, and stir until all flour lumps are blended.

3. Slowly add milk and Parmesan cheese, and increase heat to medium-high. Cook, stirring constantly, for 3 to 5 minutes.

4. Mix in garlic powder, pepper, and spinach. Remove from heat when creamy.

5. Toss spinach sauce with drained pasta and shrimp. Serve with a colorful salad.

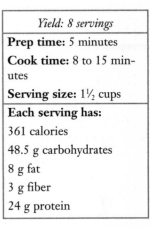 **Tummy Trouble**

Traditionally, alfredo sauce made with cream is loaded with fat and lactose and can be a sure-bet trigger for IBS. But this version, made with reduced-lactose low-fat milk, is much easier for the IBS body to tolerate.

Asian Sesame Noodles

These Asian-style noodles are mixed with colorful vegetables and enveloped in a sweet-and-sour dressing.

Yield: 6 servings
Prep time: 15 minutes
Cook time: 8 to 15 minutes
Serving size: 1½ cups
Each serving has:
400 calories
54 g carbohydrates
15.5 g fat
5 g fiber
9 g protein

1 (12-oz.) pkg. rice spaghetti

¼ cup orange juice

2 TB. reduced-sodium tamari or soy sauce

1 TB. sesame oil

2 TB. vegetable oil

2 tsp. fresh ginger, minced

2 tsp. brown sugar, firmly packed

⅓ cup crunchy peanut butter

¼ tsp. crushed red pepper flakes

1½ cups shredded carrots (2 large carrots)

1 medium red bell pepper, ribs and seeds removed, and cut into strips

1½ cups snow peas, ends trimmed and cut in half

2 TB. sesame seeds

½ cup chopped fresh cilantro (optional)

1. Cook pasta according to package directions.

2. Meanwhile, in a small bowl, whisk together orange juice, tamari, sesame oil, vegetable oil, ginger, brown sugar, peanut butter, and red pepper flakes.

3. In a medium serving dish, add carrots, red bell pepper, and snow peas.

4. Drain and rinse pasta, and immediately toss over vegetables, allowing the heat from pasta to quick-steam vegetables. Drizzle dressing over pasta and vegetables, and mix to blend.

5. Garnish with sesame seeds and cilantro (if using). Enjoy warm.

Digestibles

You can find rice spaghetti in health food stores or in the gluten-free sections of some markets. Rice pasta is very similar in taste and texture to traditional wheat pasta. Use plenty of water to cook rice pasta, and add a splash of oil to the water to prevent the rice pasta from becoming sticky. Because it's free of fructans, rice pasta may be better tolerated in the IBS body.

American Chop Suey

This hearty pasta dish will soon become a family favorite. It can be doubled easily when you need to feed a crowd.

1 lb. elbow macaroni

1 lb. 90-percent-extra-lean ground beef

1 (14.5-oz.) can diced tomatoes, drained

1 cup tomato sauce or jarred spaghetti sauce

1 tsp. Italian seasoning

½ tsp. garlic salt

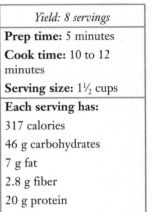

Yield: 8 servings
Prep time: 5 minutes
Cook time: 10 to 12 minutes
Serving size: 1½ cups
Each serving has:
317 calories
46 g carbohydrates
7 g fat
2.8 g fiber
20 g protein

1. Cook pasta according to package directions. Drain, rinse, and keep warm.

2. Meanwhile, in a large, nonstick skillet over medium heat, brown ground beef. Cook, stirring, for 8 to 10 minutes. Drain any excess fat from meat.

3. Add diced tomatoes, tomato sauce, Italian seasoning, and garlic salt, and stir to combine.

4. In a medium serving bowl, add warm pasta, and stir in meat mixture. Serve with a garden salad.

Gut Facts _____

Feel free to substitute ground turkey or ground chicken breast for an even lower-fat version of this recipe.

Patsy's Macaroni and Cheese

Rethink the traditional mac 'n' cheese! You'll love every creamy bite of this reinvented pasta favorite. *(Reprinted with permission from IBSFree.net by Patsy Catsos, R.D.)*

Yield: 4 servings
Prep time: 10 to 15 minutes
Cook time: 25 minutes
Serving size: 1 cup
Each serving has:
507 calories
55 g carbohydrates
21 g fat
6 g fiber
22 g protein

2 cups quinoa or corn pasta

2 TB. cornstarch

½ tsp. dry mustard

½ tsp. salt

¼ tsp. freshly ground black pepper

1¾ cups reduced-lactose low-fat milk

2 cups cheddar cheese, grated

½ tsp. crushed red pepper flakes

½ cup crumbled potato chips, corn chips, or gluten-free breadcrumbs

1. Preheat the oven to 350°F. Spray 9×9 baking dish with nonstick cooking spray.

2. Cook pasta according to package directions until slightly undercooked (or al dente) and soft but with a firm texture. Drain, rinse, and keep warm.

3. Meanwhile, in a medium saucepan over medium heat, combine cornstarch, dry mustard, salt, pepper, and milk, and stir until smooth. Continue cooking for 3 to 5 minutes or until boiling.

4. Add cheese and red pepper flakes while stirring constantly. Remove from heat.

5. Add warm pasta to cheese sauce, and place in the prepared baking dish. Sprinkle crumbled chips over top of casserole, and bake, uncovered, for 25 minutes or until crumbs are lightly browned on top.

Gut Facts

Cheddar cheese and lactose-free milk make this pasta tolerable for those with lactose intolerance. Substituting a fructan-free alternative for the wheat pasta makes this dish even more belly-friendly.

Portobello Mushroom Pasta

Hearty portobello mushrooms lend a rich, beefy taste to this savory pasta dish.

1 lb. whole-wheat, corn, or rice ziti or penne pasta

2 TB. butter or trans-fat-free margarine

¼ cup olive or vegetable oil

1 clove garlic, sliced in thirds

1 tsp. onion powder

1 tsp. Italian seasoning

1 (14.5-oz.) can low-sodium fat-free chicken broth

½ cup dry white wine

6 medium portobello mushrooms, cleaned and sliced

1 medium red bell pepper, ribs and seeds removed, and cut into strips

3 cups fresh spinach, stems removed and washed

Yield: 8 servings
Prep time: 8 to 15 minutes
Cook time: 8 minutes
Serving size: 1½ cups
Each serving has:
337 calories
48 g carbohydrates
11 g fat
5 g fiber
11 g protein

1. Cook pasta according to package directions. Drain, rinse, and keep warm.

2. Meanwhile, in a large skillet over low heat, add butter, olive oil, and garlic. Sauté for 1 or 2 minutes or until garlic is fragrant. Remove and discard garlic.

3. Add onion powder, Italian seasoning, chicken broth, and white wine to the skillet. Increase heat to medium-high, and cook, stirring gently, for 2 minutes.

4. Add mushrooms and red bell pepper, and cook for 2 or 3 more minutes. Add spinach, and remove from heat. Spinach will wilt quickly. Stir and then toss with warm pasta.

 Digestibles

To clean mushrooms, gently wipe them with a damp cloth or soft brush, rather than submerse them in water. This helps the mushrooms maintain their light texture and not get waterlogged.

Lemony Orzo with Pine Nuts, Tomatoes, Basil, and Garlic

Your first taste of this lemony-garlicy dish will bring you right to the Mediterranean Sea.

Yield: 5 servings
Prep time: 5 minutes
Cook time: 8 to 15 minutes
Serving size: 1 cup
Each serving has:
357 calories
37 g carbohydrates
20 g fat
2.8 g fiber
8 g protein

1⅓ **cups** *orzo* **pasta**

¼ **cup olive or vegetable oil**

½ **cup pine nuts**

2 cloves garlic, cut in half

2 cups grape tomatoes, cut in half

2 TB. freshly squeezed lemon juice (1 lemon)

2 TB. fresh basil, cut into fine strips

1. In a large saucepan, cook pasta according to package directions.

2. Meanwhile, in a medium skillet over medium-low heat, add olive oil, pine nuts, and garlic. Sauté, stirring frequently, for 1 minute or until garlic sizzles and pine nuts are lightly brown. Remove from heat, discard garlic, and set skillet aside.

3. In a medium serving bowl, add tomatoes. Drain pasta, rinse under warm water, and add immediately to tomatoes while hot to steam them. Drizzle with pine nut–oil mixture. Add lemon juice, and gently stir. Garnish with fresh basil, and serve.

Wellness Words

> **Orzo** is a rice-shape pasta often used in hearty soups. It's also wonderful in cold and hot pasta dishes.

The Original Cheese Pizza

You'll be hard-pressed to find anyone who doesn't love this tomato and cheesy pizza! It's the true original.

2 tsp. finely ground cornmeal	**1 cup marinara sauce (your favorite)**
1 TB. olive or vegetable oil	
1 pkg. frozen white, whole-wheat, or herb pizza dough, defrosted	**1 cup part-skim mozzarella cheese**

Yield: 8 pizza squares
Prep time: 10 minutes
Cook time: 10 to 15 minutes
Serving size: 1 square
Each serving has:
254 calories
40 g carbohydrates
4 g fat
4.6 g fiber
11 g protein

1. Preheat the oven to 400°F. Spray an 11×15-inch jelly-roll pan with nonstick cooking spray, and evenly sprinkle with cornmeal.

2. Drizzle olive oil in the bottom of a shallow bowl, and add pizza dough. Let sit for 5 minutes, turn dough over just to cover other side of dough with oil.

3. Remove dough from the bowl, and, over the sink, gently stretch dough with your hands into the shape of the jelly-roll pan, moving dough around in your hands to stretch two sides at a time. Place stretched pizza dough on the prepared jelly-roll pan. If it tries to retract, gently pull it back to shape to fit the pan.

4. Pour marinara sauce over dough, evenly spreading it out with the back of a spoon or a pastry brush. Sprinkle evenly with mozzarella cheese. Bake on the bottom rack for 10 to 15 minutes or until crust is golden brown on bottom. Enjoy pizza with a colorful salad.

Variation: For a heartier version, make this a **Roasted Tricolor Pepper Pizza.** Prior to preparing pizza, seed and chop red, yellow, and green bell peppers into strips. Place on a cookie sheet, drizzle with 1 tablespoon olive or vegetable oil, and bake at 400°F for 15 minutes. Remove and place peppers on top of uncooked cheese pizza, and bake as directed.

Gut Facts

Look for pre-made pizza dough in the bakery or freezer section of your grocery store. Whole-grain dough offers a high-fiber and more nutrient-rich option.

BLT Pizza

There's nothing quite like the bacon, lettuce, and tomato trio on top of freshly baked dough!

Yield: *8 pieces*
Prep time: 15 minutes
Cook time: 10 to 15 minutes
Serving size: 1 pizza square
Each serving has:
289 calories
38 g carbohydrates
11 g fat
4.4 g fiber
10 g protein

2 tsp. finely ground cornmeal

2 TB. olive or vegetable oil

1 pkg. frozen white or whole-wheat pizza dough, defrosted

$\frac{1}{4}$ cup grated Parmesan cheese

$\frac{1}{4}$ tsp. freshly ground black pepper

$\frac{1}{3}$ medium head iceberg lettuce, finely shredded

$\frac{1}{4}$ cup reduced-fat mayonnaise

8 slices turkey bacon, cooked and cut into bite-size chunks

$1\frac{1}{2}$ cups grape tomatoes, cut in half

1. Preheat the oven to 400°F. Spray an 11×15-inch jelly-roll pan with nonstick cooking spray, and evenly sprinkle with cornmeal.

2. Drizzle 1 tablespoon olive oil in the bottom of a shallow bowl, and add pizza dough. Let sit for 5 minutes, and turn dough over, just to cover other side of dough with oil.

3. Remove dough from the bowl, and, over the sink, gently stretch dough with your hands into the shape of the jelly-roll pan, moving dough around in your hands to stretch two sides at a time. Place stretched pizza dough on the prepared jelly-roll pan. If it tries to retract, gently pull it back to shape to fit the pan.

4. Drizzle pizza with remaining 1 tablespoon olive oil, and sprinkle evenly with Parmesan cheese and pepper. Bake on the bottom rack for 10 to 15 minutes or until crust is golden brown on bottom. Remove from the oven.

5. In a medium bowl, gently mix lettuce with mayonnaise. Top pizza with lettuce mixture, followed by bacon, followed by tomatoes. Cut into 8 pieces, and serve.

Gut Facts

Uncured bacon is a more healthful alternative to the traditionally sodium nitrite–cured bacon linked with increased risk of cancer.

Variation: For the Mexican food lovers in your life, consider making this a **Mexican Pizza.** Layer a plain baked pizza crust with 1 pound cooked and drained extra-lean ground beef, followed by 1 cup grated cheddar cheese. For extra zip, garnish with shredded iceberg lettuce, diced tomatoes, 1 cup broken tortilla chips, and possibly a taste of reduced-fat sour cream. If you and your belly don't mind a bit of heat, add a sprinkle or two of hot sauce!

Arugula and Prosciutto Pizza

Tangy and salty meats complement the peppery herbs in this Italian favorite.

2 tsp. finely ground cornmeal

4 TB. vegetable oil

1 pkg. frozen white or whole-wheat pizza dough, defrosted

¼ tsp. freshly ground black pepper

2 cups baby arugula

1 TB. freshly squeezed lemon juice (1 lemon)

½ cup flaked Parmesan cheese

3 thin slices prosciutto, cut into bite-size pieces

Yield: 8 pieces
Prep time: 10 minutes
Cook time: 10 to 15 minutes
Serving size: 1 square
Each serving has:
273 calories
36 g carbohydrates
10 g fat
4 g fiber
10 g protein

1. Preheat the oven to 400°F. Spray an 11×15-inch jelly-roll pan with nonstick cooking spray, and evenly sprinkle with cornmeal.

2. Drizzle 1 tablespoon vegetable oil in the bottom of a shallow bowl, and add pizza dough. Let sit for 5 minutes, turn dough over just to cover other side of dough with oil.

3. Remove dough from the bowl, and, over the sink, gently stretch dough with your hands into the shape of the jelly-roll pan, moving dough around in your hands to stretch two sides at a time. Place stretched pizza dough on the prepared jelly-roll pan. If it tries to retract, gently pull it back to shape to fit the pan.

5. Drizzle pizza with 1 tablespoon vegetable oil, and sprinkle evenly with pepper. Bake on the bottom rack for 10 to 15 minutes or until crust is golden brown on bottom. Remove from the oven.

6. In a medium bowl, combine arugula, lemon juice, remaining 2 tablespoons vegetable oil, and Parmesan cheese. Evenly disperse arugula mixture over pizza, and top with prosciutto pieces.

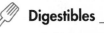 **Digestibles**

For this pizza, slice the prosciutto paper thin. Its salty taste can be overpowering if overused. Prosciutto is a specialty ham from Italy that's air cured.

Ground Beef Tostado Pizza

What happens when Italy meets Mexico? Here's the answer! This pizza is like an open-faced taco.

Yield: 6 servings
Prep time: 20 minutes
Cook time: 10 minutes
Serving size: 2 tostado pizzas
Each serving has:
321 calories
16 g carbohydrates
18 g fat
1 g fiber
22 g protein

1 lb. 90-percent-extra-lean ground beef

2 tsp. chili powder

1 tsp. ground cumin

½ tsp. garlic powder

1 (14.5-oz.) can diced tomatoes, drained

12 tostado shells

1 cup grated sharp or low-fat cheddar cheese

1. Preheat the oven to 350°F.

2. In a large, nonstick skillet over medium heat, add ground beef and cook, crumbling and stirring, for 5 to 10 minutes. Drain excess fat from meat, and add chili powder, cumin, garlic powder, and diced tomatoes to the skillet. Reduce heat to low, and simmer for 5 to 10 minutes.

3. On a large cookie sheet, spread out 12 tostado shells. Divide meat mixture evenly among tostado shells. Sprinkle cheddar cheese evenly over meat mixture. Bake for 10 minutes. Enjoy with a garden salad.

Digestibles

Instead of buying premade taco seasoning packets, try substituting 1 tablespoon chili powder, 1 teaspoon ground cumin, and ½ teaspoon garlic or onion salt. This DIY mix saves you a few pennies and offers fewer additives and preservatives. Many of the commercial seasoning packets contain hidden gluten, too.

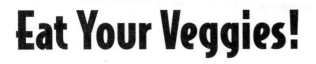

Chapter

19

Eat Your Veggies!

In This Chapter

- ◆ Eating your way through the vegetable garden
- ◆ Remarkable roasted vegetables
- ◆ Scrumptious veggie stir-fries, medleys, and purées
- ◆ Pleasing potato provisions

Experts recommend eating 5 to 9 servings of fruits and vegetables a day for good health. We know a diet rich in fruits and vegetables is a key ingredient to good health. Experts have linked lowered risk of stroke; heart disease; and cancers of the mouth, stomach, and colon with adequate produce in the diet. Vegetables rich in potassium appear to also reduce risk for kidney stones and keep bones healthy. So are you meeting your daily quota of all-important fruits and vegetables?

In this chapter, I give you veggies galore prepared in so many tantalizing new ways. You may find that your veggie-phobic friends or family turn a new leaf and start gobbling up these nutritional superstars. Including a colorful veggie or two at every meal and snack time is an easy way to maximize your intake.

Now get going, get healthy, and make some vegetables!

Singapore Stir-Fry

This delightfully aromatic Asian-inspired vegetable dish cooks in a flash.

Yield: 6 servings
Prep time: 10 minutes
Cook time: 8 to 10 minutes
Serving size: 1 cup
Each serving has:
93 calories
5 g carbohydrates
7 g fat
2 g fiber
2.3 g protein

2 TB. peanut or vegetable oil

2 cups button mushrooms, cleaned and sliced thin

2 medium carrots, peeled and cut on diagonal into thin rounds

1 medium red bell pepper, ribs and seeds removed, and cut into thin strips

1 cup snow peas, ends trimmed

2 TB. reduced-sodium tamari or soy sauce

1 tsp. fresh ginger, minced

1 tsp. garlic powder

1 tsp. *sesame oil*

2 TB. sesame seeds

1. In a large skillet over medium heat, combine peanut oil, mushrooms, carrots, and red bell pepper. Cook for 3 to 5 minutes.

2. Add snow peas, reduce heat to low, and cook for 1 more minute.

3. In a small bowl, whisk together tamari, ginger, garlic powder, and sesame oil. Drizzle over vegetables in the skillet, and remove the skillet from heat.

4. In a small skillet over medium heat, add sesame seeds. Toast for about 2 minutes or until sesame seeds are fragrant and caramel colored. Garnish vegetables with toasted sesame seeds.

Wellness Words

Sesame oil infuses a recipe with a nutty flavor reminiscent of many Asian dishes. It may lower blood pressure, is a good source of heart-healthy monounsaturated fats, and is rich in disease-fighting antioxidants—plus it tastes really good! Look for it in the Asian or international section of most grocery stores.

Peppers and Mushroom Medley

This savory wine-, butter-, and herb-infused medley will spruce up any meal.

6 cups assorted button and *portobello* mushrooms, sliced

1 medium red bell pepper, ribs and seeds removed, and sliced into thin strips

2 TB. olive or vegetable oil

⅓ cup dry white wine

1 TB. butter

2 TB. chopped fresh parsley

2 tsp. chopped fresh thyme

¼ tsp. onion salt

¼ tsp. freshly ground black pepper

Yield: 6 servings
Prep time: 10 minutes
Cook time: 4 or 5 minutes
Serving size: ½ cup
Each serving has:
96 calories
5 g carbohydrates
7 g fat
1.5 g fiber
2 g protein

1. In a large skillet over medium heat, add mushrooms, red bell pepper, and olive oil. Sauté for 2 or 3 minutes or until peppers are soft and mushrooms are golden brown. Drain any extra liquid.

2. Add white wine, reduce heat to low, and simmer for 3 minutes.

3. Add butter, parsley, thyme, onion salt, and pepper, and gently stir. Enjoy over grilled fish or as a side to your favorite meatloaf recipe.

 Wellness Words

Portobello mushrooms are grown-up crimini mushrooms. Large portobellos are meaty and can be used as a sandwich filler. They're also low in fat and rich in fiber.

Vegetable Chop Suey

There's lots of veggie crunch in this taste-of-Asia side dish.

Yield: 8 servings
Prep time: 10 to 15 minutes
Cook time: 10 minutes
Serving size: 1 cup
Each serving has:
78 calories
9 g carbohydrates
3.5 g fat
2 g fiber
3 g protein

2 TB. peanut or vegetable oil

4 medium carrots, peeled and sliced into thin rounds

1 medium red bell pepper, ribs and seeds removed, and cut into ¼-in. strips

5 TB. reduced-sodium tamari or soy sauce

2 TB. cornstarch

5 medium stalks celery, sliced

2 cups button mushrooms, sliced

2 cups bean sprouts

1. In a large skillet over medium-low heat, combine peanut oil, carrots, and red bell pepper, and cook, stirring, for 3 to 5 minutes.

2. In a small bowl, whisk together tamari and cornstarch, and pour over carrots.

3. Add celery, mushrooms, and bean sprouts, cover, and reduce heat to low. Cook, stirring occasionally, for 5 more minutes. Enjoy with brown rice and grilled seafood.

Gut Facts

Chop suey is an American- and Chinese-influenced dish typically made with vegetables, especially bean sprouts, and bite-size meats in a savory, Asian-style sauce.

Roasted Vegetables

This burst of colorful, garlic-infused veggies will delight your palate.

1 medium zucchini, skin on and sliced into $\frac{1}{2}$-in. rounds

1 medium yellow squash, skin on and sliced into $\frac{1}{2}$-in. rounds

1 medium orange bell pepper, ribs and seeds removed, and cut into strips

1 medium red bell pepper, ribs and seeds removed, and cut into strips

$\frac{1}{4}$ cup pine nuts

2 TB. olive or vegetable oil

1 tsp. garlic salt

$\frac{1}{2}$ tsp. freshly ground black pepper

Yield: 8 cups
Prep time: 10 to 15 minutes
Cook time: 15 to 20 minutes
Serving size: 1 cup
Each serving has:
77 calories
3.8 g carbohydrates
6.5 g fat
1.3 g fiber
1 g protein

1. Preheat the oven to 400°F. Spray a cookie sheet with nonstick cooking spray.

2. In a large bowl, combine zucchini, yellow squash, orange bell pepper, red bell pepper, pine nuts, and olive oil. Stir to evenly coat.

3. Spread vegetables and pine nuts in even layer on the prepared cookie sheet. Sprinkle with garlic salt and pepper.

4. Bake on the middle rack for 10 minutes. Using a spatula, turn vegetables over and cook for 5 to 10 more minutes. Enjoy these wonderfully roasted vegetables over pasta or as a side dish.

Gut Facts

Bell peppers are a great source of vitamin C. Red bell peppers also provide lutein and zeaxanthin, two phytochemicals that have been found to reduce the risk of macular degeneration, the main cause of blindness in the elderly.

Yellow Summer Squash with Bacon

The sweet squash in this quick-fix dish pairs well with the salty bacon.

Yield: 6 servings
Prep time: 5 minutes
Cook time: 8 to 10 minutes
Serving size: 1 cup
Each serving has:
55 calories
2 g carbohydrates
4 g fat
.6 g fiber
2 g protein

2 medium or large summer squashes, skin on and cut into rounds

4 strips turkey bacon, cut into bite-size pieces

1 TB. olive or vegetable oil

¼ tsp. freshly ground black pepper

1. In a large skillet over medium heat, add squash, bacon, and olive oil. Cook for 8 to 10 minutes, stirring bacon and flipping over squash rounds.

2. Garnish with freshly ground pepper, and serve with your favorite grilled fish or beef dish.

Gut Facts

Summer squash has a mild flavor and is a good source of vitamin C.

Stuffed Tomatoes

These cheesy tomatoes are as pretty as they are tasty!

3 large tomatoes

½ cup chopped fresh parsley

½ cup plain or Italian-style breadcrumbs

½ tsp. garlic salt

2 TB. olive oil

1 TB. butter, melted

⅓ cup grated Parmesan cheese

Yield: 6 servings
Prep time: 10 minutes
Cook time: 15 to 20 minutes
Serving size: ½ tomato
Each serving has:
136 calories
10.5 g carbohydrates
8.6 g fat
1.6 g fiber
4.2 g protein

1. Preheat the oven to 350°F.

2. Cut tomatoes in half. Scoop out seeds and flesh and place in a small mixing bowl.

3. Add parsley, breadcrumbs, garlic salt, olive oil, and melted butter, and stir to combine.

4. Fill tomato halves with breadcrumb mixture and then evenly sprinkle Parmesan cheese over each. Bake for 15 to 20 minutes or until heated through and slightly soft.

 Digestibles _____

This recipe is a great way to use up all those red, ripe tomatoes from your garden before they go bad. Tomatoes are a terrific source of potassium and vitamin C.

Sweet Potato and Carrot Purée

This recipe is creamy with a hint of spice. Enjoy it alongside a serving of roasted chicken for a truly comforting meal. *(Adapted and reprinted with permission from IBSFree.net by Patsy Catsos, R.D.)*

Yield: 7 servings
Prep time: 10 minutes
Cook time: 60 minutes
Serving size: 1 cup
Each serving has:
133 calories
20 g carbohydrates
5 g fat
3.4 g fiber
2 g protein

Gut Facts

Sweet potatoes and carrots provide your body with vitamin A, an essential nutrient for eye health.

2 large sweet potatoes	$\frac{1}{2}$ cup reduced-lactose skim milk
6 medium carrots, peeled and sliced	$\frac{1}{2}$ tsp. freshly grated nutmeg
3 TB. butter	Dash cayenne (optional)
1 TB. sugar	Salt
2 cups water	Freshly ground black pepper

1. Preheat the oven to 375°F.

2. Poke sweet potatoes with a knife 3 or 4 times, and place on the middle oven rack. Bake for 45 to 60 minutes or until fork-tender. Set aside to cool.

3. In a medium-large saucepan over medium-high heat, add carrots, butter, sugar, and water. Bring to a boil, reduce heat to medium-low, and cook for about 15 minutes or until water is absorbed. Be careful not to burn carrots.

4. Scrape sweet potato flesh into the saucepan. Add milk, grated nutmeg, and cayenne (if using), and mix well. Purée mixture in a blender or a food processor fitted with a metal blade, or mash with a potato masher right in the saucepan for a chunkier texture. Season with salt and pepper, and serve warm.

Steamed Broccoli with Sesame Dressing

A wonderful light sauce and nutty sesame seeds are the perfect complement to the calcium-rich broccoli.

4 cups broccoli florets

2 TB. reduced-sodium tamari or soy sauce

1 TB. freshly squeezed lemon juice (½ lemon)

½ tsp. sesame oil

1 tsp. garlic powder

2 TB. sesame seeds, toasted

Yield: 4 servings
Prep time: 5 minutes
Cook time: 5 or 6 minutes
Serving size: 1 cup
Each serving has:
42 calories
7 g carbohydrates
.8 g fat
2.4 g fiber
3 g protein

1. In steamer over high heat, steam broccoli for 5 or 6 minutes or until desired texture. If you don't have a steamer, place ¾ cup water in a medium-large saucepan over high heat. Bring to a boil, and carefully add broccoli. Cook for 1 or 2 minutes, stirring occasionally. Turn off heat, cover pan, and let sit for 2 or 3 minutes. Broccoli is done when it becomes darker in color and is fork-tender. Place broccoli in a serving bowl.

2. In a small bowl, whisk together tamari, lemon juice, sesame oil, and garlic powder, and immediately drizzle over broccoli. Garnish with toasted sesame seeds.

Digestibles

To toast sesame seeds, place them in a small skillet over medium heat. Occasionally stir or shake the pan to move the seeds, cooking for about 2 minutes or until the seeds are caramel-colored. Remove the seeds from the pan immediately to stop the cooking process.

Ann's Cumin Corn with Cilantro

Subtle notes of Indian spices infuse this delicious corn dish. Dr. Ann, from my Boston office, inspired this dish.

Yield: 8 servings
Prep time: 5 minutes
Cook time: 5 to 10 minutes
Serving size: $\frac{1}{2}$ cup
Each serving has:
103 calories
17 g carbohydrates
4 g fat
2 g fiber
1.5 g protein

2 TB. olive or vegetable oil

4 cups frozen corn

1 tsp. *turmeric*

1 tsp. ground cumin

$\frac{1}{4}$ tsp. salt

2 TB. chopped fresh cilantro

1. In a large skillet over medium heat, heat olive oil. Add corn, turmeric, cumin, and salt. Cook, stirring occasionally, for 5 to 10 minutes.

2. Sprinkle with cilantro, and serve warm as a side dish.

Wellness Words

Turmeric is a bright-yellow spice often used in Indian cooking. Studies have suggested that the chemical curcumin, found in turmeric, may have anti-inflammatory and anticancer properties.

Glazed Carrots

Even kids will like these delightfully sweet orange veggies.

6 to 8 medium carrots, peeled and sliced into thin rounds (3 cups)

2 cups water

1 TB. butter

1 TB. olive oil

¼ cup firmly packed brown sugar, or to taste

2 TB. dry mustard

¼ tsp. salt

1 TB. chopped fresh parsley

Yield: 6 servings
Prep time: 5 minutes
Cook time: 8 minutes
Serving size: ½ cup
Each serving has:
97 calories
15 g carbohydrates
4.4 g fat
1.8 g fiber
.2 g protein

1. In a large skillet over medium heat, combine carrots and water. Cook for 5 minutes, drain off any remaining water, and remove carrots to a serving dish.

2. Dry the skillet, and set over medium heat. Add butter and olive oil, and stir in brown sugar, dry mustard, and salt. Cook for 1 minute.

3. Add carrots back to the skillet, and cook for 1 or 2 more minutes. Remove from heat, garnish with parsley, and serve.

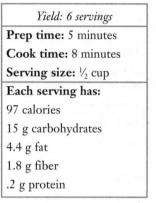 **Digestibles** _____

Carrots are one root vegetable, but how familiar are you with other, less famous roots like rutabaga, turnip, parsnip, and beets? Root vegetables grow underground and act as the stem or root of a plant. They pull nutrients from the nutrient-rich soil as they ripen and are often ready for harvest in the early fall. Root vegetables are jammed-pack with fiber; vitamins A, B, C; and folic acid.

Smashed Potatoes

These quick-fix potatoes give you a boost of fiber, thanks to the intact skins. These potatoes really stick to your ribs.

Yield: 6 servings
Prep time: 10 minutes
Cook time: 15 to 20 minutes
Serving size: ½ cup
Each serving has:
183 calories
33.6 g carbohydrates
4 g fat
3.5 g fiber
4 g protein

6 medium red-skinned potatoes, skin on, scrubbed, and quartered

1 clove garlic

⅓ cup low-sodium fat-free chicken broth

2 TB. butter or trans-fat-free margarine

½ tsp. garlic salt

1. In a large stockpot over high heat, add potatoes and garlic, and fill ¾ full of water. Bring to a boil, and cook potatoes for about 15 to 20 minutes or until fork-tender.

2. Drain water from potatoes, and carefully remove garlic clove with a fork.

3. Return the pot to the stove. Reduce heat to low, and add chicken broth, butter, and garlic salt. Mash with a potato masher for about 1 or 2 minutes or until creamy. Enjoy with Turkey Tenderloin (recipe in Chapter 17).

Gut Facts

Potatoes are a rich source of potassium, vitamin C, and fiber, particularly when you eat the skin. Potatoes are a fat- and sodium-free food, too.

Sweet Potato Fries

Sweet and crunchy, these baked sweet potato fries are a healthier alternative to traditional fried french fries!

2 TB. olive or vegetable oil	½ tsp. freshly ground black pepper
2 large sweet potatoes, skin on and scrubbed	½ tsp. paprika
1 tsp. garlic salt	

1. Preheat the oven to 400°F.

2. Drizzle olive oil over an 11×15-inch jelly-roll pan.

3. Cut sweet potatoes into steak-fry shape and add to the pre-pared jelly-roll pan, moving them around with your fingers to ensure all potatoes are coated with oil.

4. In a small bowl, mix together garlic salt, pepper, and paprika, and sprinkle over potatoes.

5. Bake for 20 to 30 minutes, turning with spatula midway through cooking time, or until potatoes are fork-tender and browned.

Yield: 4 servings
Prep time: 5 to 10 minutes
Cook time: 25 to 30 minutes
Serving size: ¼ batch
Each serving has:
146 calories
19.5 g carbohydrates
7 g fat
3 g fiber
1.5 g protein

Gut Facts

Sweet potatoes are loaded with carotenoids. Carotenoids are plant pigments that provide color to deep-green, yellow, orange, and red plant foods. The most widely studied carotenoid is beta-carotene. Carotenoids are believed to help maintain eye health and minimize cancer risk when consumed from plant foods versus taken in supplement form.

Brennan's Favorite Home Fries

Crispy and seasoned just right, these potatoes are a big hit every time!

Yield: 6 servings
Prep time: 5 minutes
Cook time: 10 minutes
Serving size: 1 cup
Each serving has:
186 calories
34 g carbohydrates
4 g fat
3.6 g fiber
4 g protein

6 medium red-skinned potatoes, skin on, and chopped into bite-size chunks

1 TB. olive or vegetable oil

1 TB. butter

1 tsp. onion salt

¼ tsp. *paprika*

¼ tsp. freshly ground black pepper

1. In a large skillet over medium heat, combine potatoes with olive oil and butter.

2. Sprinkle potatoes with onion salt, paprika, and pepper. Using a spatula, flip potatoes over and scrape any residual potato off the bottom of the pan. Cook for about 10 minutes or until potatoes are browned, fork-tender and have a slight crispy exterior.

Wellness Words

Paprika is a red spice made from dried peppers. A small amount of paprika adds a touch of color and spice to your favorite dip, potato, fish, and chicken recipes. For a smoky flavor, try smoked Spanish paprika.

Potato Pancakes

Kids and adults alike love the idea of eating these buttery potatoes in pancake form!

3 medium Yukon gold potatoes, peeled and grated

½ tsp. onion salt

½ tsp. onion powder

1 tsp. dried parsley

2 large eggs, beaten

2 TB. flour

3 TB. olive or vegetable oil

Yield: 8 pancakes
Prep time: 15 minutes
Cook time: 12 to 15 minutes
Serving size: 1 pancake
Each serving has:
120 calories
14 g carbohydrates
6 g fat
1.2 g fiber
3 g protein

1. In a medium bowl, combine potatoes, onion salt, onion powder, parsley, eggs, and flour.

2. In a large, nonstick skillet over medium-high heat, add 2 tablespoons olive oil. Using a ⅓-cup measure, form a potato pancake patty, and place in the hot skillet. Repeat until you have 4 pancakes in the skillet. Flatten with a spatula, and cook for 3 minutes per side. When pancakes are cooked, remove from the skillet and keep warm.

3. Repeat with remaining potatoes, adding remaining 1 tablespoon olive oil to the skillet as necessary. Serve immediately, perhaps with the Marinated Flank Steak with Soy Sauce and Shallots (recipe in Chapter 16).

 Digestibles

Yukon gold potatoes are a sweet and buttery-tasting potato that retain their golden color even after they're cooked. To grate, you can use either a box grater or a food processor fitted with a grating blade.

Chapter 20

Rich Rice and Grains

In This Chapter

◆ Hearty and satisfying grains

◆ Risotto with a twist

◆ Out-of-the-typical-box whole grains

When you're looking for a hearty dish that settles nicely in your belly, turn to the rice and grain dishes in this chapter. Whole grains are a terrific source of complex carbohydrates, key nutrients that provide your body with needed energy, vitamins, and minerals. Not to mention they contain a hefty dose of phytochemicals, important disease-fighting plant substances.

Whole grains offer more bang for their buck because they contain all parts of the grain. The major parts of whole grains include the bran, germ, and endosperm. The bran contains most of the fiber, while the germ is a terrific source of vitamins and minerals. The endosperm makes up the majority of the grain and provides some protein. Refined grains, stripped of the germ and bran until they're mostly the starchy endosperm, have diminished nutrients.

Be adventurous with whole grains, and boost your intake of zinc, copper, vitamin E, magnesium, and B vitamins! The wide range of whole-grain recipes in this chapter is a great place to start!

Reach for Rice (and Risotto)

More rice varieties are available than there are days in the week. Some of my favorites are wild rice, jasmine, brown, and especially Chinese black rice. Rice is a great wheat-free grain option that can be spruced up in so many ways.

Arborio rice is the key ingredient in making classic Italian risotto. This high-starch, short-grained rice makes a creamy dish, thanks to the extra starch this rice releases as it cooks. Mix in a little broth, and you've created a velvety treat. To me, nothing says comfort food more than risotto.

Not Your Average Grains

There's a whole world of grains available for the taking. Look around your local health store, food co-op, or international market, and you'll see what I mean. If you haven't ventured beyond rice, wheat, and corn, this will be an interesting journey for you!

Many experts believe that rotating our grains is more healthful than simply saturating our body with the same grains daily. So try to step outside of your grain box and enjoy millet, kasha, or even quinoa, for starters. In this chapter, you'll find some interesting ways to try these less-common grains while enhancing your nutrient repertoire.

Yes, you'll impress your friends with these alternative grains, but you'll also bolster your protein intake with protein-rich quinoa, add some fiber with kasha, or kick up your iron intake with millet. Whole grains in general are rich in magnesium and B vitamins, too!

Asian Flare Faux Fried Rice

Toasted sesame and citrus hints of coriander infuse this lower-fat version of fried rice.

1 TB. olive or vegetable oil

2 tsp. sesame oil

1 cup bean sprouts

1 cup snow peas, ends trimmed and cut in half on the diagonal

1 medium red bell pepper, ribs and seeds removed, and cut into bite-size pieces

1 medium carrot, peeled and sliced into thin rounds

2 cups cooked brown rice

1 tsp. coriander

2 TB. reduced-sodium tamari or soy sauce

Yields: 4 servings
Prep time: 5 to 10 minutes
Cook time: 7 to 9 minutes
Serving size: 1 cup
Each serving has:
204 calories
31 g carbohydrates
6 g fat
4 g fiber
5.5 g protein

1. In a large skillet over medium heat, combine olive oil, sesame oil, bean sprouts, snow peas, red bell pepper, and carrots. Cook for 5 minutes.

2. Add rice, and stir gently. Add coriander and drizzle with tamari, and let vegetables steam lightly for 2 to 4 more minutes. Serve with a side of grilled chicken or fish.

Digestibles

More and more brands of microwaveable brown rice are available in the freezer section of many grocery stores. In just a few minutes, you can enjoy this hearty rice alone or dressed up with a few ingredients, such as in this recipe.

Not-from-a-Box Rice Pilaf

Throw out the boxed rice pilaf, and try this delightfully savory homemade version!

Yield: 4 cups
Prep time: 5 to 10 minutes
Cook time: 20 to 25 minutes
Serving size: 1 cup
Each serving has:
272 calories
44 g carbohydrates
8 g fat
4 g fiber
5 g protein

1 TB. butter or trans-fat-free margarine

1 TB. vegetable oil

½ cup whole-wheat angel hair pasta, broken into 1-in. pieces

1 cup brown rice

3 cups low-sodium fat-free chicken broth

½ tsp. Bell's Seasoning or poultry seasoning

¼ tsp. freshly ground black pepper

½ tsp. onion powder

½ tsp. garlic salt

2 TB. finely chopped fresh parsley

1. In a large skillet over medium heat, add butter and vegetable oil, and heat until melted. Add angel hair pasta, and cook for 1 or 2 minutes or until golden brown.

2. Add brown rice, chicken broth, Bell's Seasoning, pepper, onion powder, and garlic salt. Increase heat to high and bring mixture to a boil. Reduce heat to low, and simmer, covered, for 20 to 25 minutes or until liquid is fully absorbed. Garnish with parsley, and serve.

🚫 Tummy Trouble

Convenience foods are traditionally high in salt, problematic if you have high blood pressure. Keeping an eye on the sodium amount in boxed versions of rice pilaf might just make you want to try this lower-sodium variety. Plus, there's the Bell's Seasoning. Bell's is a mixture of rosemary, oregano, sage, ginger, and marjoram—all fabulous spices for poultry stuffing and this tasty pilaf.

Chicken Rice Bowl

This quick-fix Asian-spiced dish is a complete meal in a bowl.

1 lb. boneless, skinless chicken breast, cut into thin strips

2 TB. peanut or vegetable oil

1 cup button mushrooms, sliced

1 medium red bell pepper, ribs and seeds removed, and cut into strips

2 TB. reduced-sodium tamari or soy sauce

¼ cup water

¼ cup orange juice

1 tsp. fresh or jarred ginger, minced

1½ TB. firmly packed brown sugar

½ tsp. garlic powder

1 TB. cornstarch

1 cup snow peas, ends trimmed

3 cups cooked brown rice, warm

Yield: 4 servings
Prep time: 10 minutes
Cook time: 10 to 14 minutes
Serving size: ¾ cup rice with ¾ cup meat and veggie topping
Each serving has:
384 calories
47 g carbohydrates
8.5 g fat
4.5 g fiber
26 g protein

1. In a large skillet over medium-high heat, combine chicken and peanut oil. Cook, stirring, for 6 to 10 minutes. Add mushrooms and red bell pepper, reduce heat to low, and gently stir for 2 or 3 minutes.

2. In a small mixing bowl, whisk together tamari, water, orange juice, ginger, brown sugar, garlic powder, and cornstarch.

3. Add soy mixture to chicken and vegetables, and increase heat to medium-high. Cook for 3 more minutes to thicken sauce. Add snow peas, cook 2 more minutes, and remove from heat.

4. Add ¾ cup brown rice to each of 4 bowls, top with chicken and vegetable mixture, and serve.

 Digestibles _____

This dish makes a great lunch to take to school or work. In fact, you can even find insulated bowl-shape containers just for this type of dish. You or your child will be the envy of the lunchroom!

Butternut Squash and Parmesan Risotto

Sweet, herb-infused roasted butternut squash is delightful in this creamy risotto.

Yield: 6 servings
Prep time: 10 to 15 minutes
Cook time: 20 to 22 minutes
Serving size: $1\frac{1}{2}$ cups
Each serving has:
353 calories
53 g carbohydrates
11 g fat
4 g fiber
8 g protein

1 (2-lb.) butternut squash, peeled and cut into 1-in. chunks

4 TB. olive or vegetable oil

1 tsp. dried rosemary

6 cups low-sodium fat-free chicken broth

$1\frac{1}{2}$ cups arborio rice

$\frac{1}{2}$ cup dry white wine

4 cups fresh baby spinach

$\frac{1}{2}$ cup reduced-lactose, low-fat milk

$\frac{1}{4}$ cup freshly grated Parmesan cheese

1. Preheat the oven to 400°F.

2. In an 11×15-inch jelly-roll pan, combine squash, 2 tablespoons olive oil, and rosemary. Bake for 20 to 30 minutes or until fork-tender. Remove from the oven, and set aside.

3. Meanwhile, in a large saucepan over medium heat, warm chicken broth.

4. While broth is heating, in a large, nonstick skillet over medium heat, combine remaining 2 tablespoons olive oil and arborio rice. Cook, stirring frequently, for 2 minutes. Add white wine to rice, and simmer for 1 more minute.

5. Using a ladle, add $\frac{1}{2}$ cup broth to rice, and stir until broth is completely absorbed. Add another $\frac{1}{2}$ cup and stir until absorbed, and repeat with rest of broth. When all broth has been added and absorbed, add spinach and reduce heat to low. Stir in milk, and cook for 1 more minute. Gently fold in squash, and garnish with Parmesan cheese. Enjoy!

Digestibles

Arborio rice becomes risotto when it's prepared. If you happen to have any leftover risotto, simply refresh it with a splash of water and reheat!

Creamy Risotto with Shredded Chicken and Broccoli

This creamy risotto is a complete meal with veggies, protein, and lots of nutritious broccoli.

6 cups low-sodium fat-free chicken broth

1½ cups arborio rice

2 TB. olive or vegetable oil

½ tsp. garlic salt

¼ tsp. freshly ground black pepper

2 cups cooked boneless, skinless chicken breast, cut into bite-size chunks

2 (10-oz.) pkgs. frozen broccoli, cooked according to pkg. directions

¼ cup grated Parmesan cheese

2 TB. finely chopped fresh parsley

Yield: 6 servings
Prep time: 5 to 10 minutes
Cook time: 20 minutes
Serving size: 1½ cups
Each serving has:
332 calories
42.5 g carbohydrates
7.5 g fat
2.4 g fiber
21 g protein

1. In a large saucepan over medium heat, warm chicken broth.

2. In a large skillet over medium-high heat, combine rice and olive oil. Cook, stirring constantly to prevent browning, for 1 or 2 minutes.

3. Using a ladle, add ½ cup broth to rice, and stir until broth is completely absorbed. Add another ½ cup and stir until absorbed, and repeat with rest of broth. When all broth has been absorbed, gently fold in cooked chicken and broccoli. Season with garlic salt and pepper, and garnish with Parmesan cheese and parsley.

Gut Facts

Broccoli is a member of the cruciferous vegetable family best known for lowering the risk of cancer. This little tree-shape vegetable is loaded with vitamins C and K. It also packs in quite a bit of calcium!

Farm Stand Vegetable Pie

The rice crust is an unusual but tasty addition to this cheese-and-veggie pie.

Yield: *6 servings*
Prep time: 15 minutes
Cook time: 33 to 35 minutes
Serving size: ⅙ pie
Each serving has:
124 calories
9 g carbohydrates
7 g fat
1 g fiber
6 g protein

¼ cup jasmine rice

2 large egg whites, lightly beaten

¼ cup grated Parmesan cheese

1 medium zucchini, skin on and sliced into thin rounds

1 medium summer squash, skin on and sliced into thin rounds

1 medium tomato, sliced into thin rounds

1 tsp. Italian seasoning

½ tsp. garlic salt

1 TB. olive or vegetable oil

½ cup grated cheddar cheese

 Digestibles

Thanks to the rice crust, this pie is a great gluten- or wheat-free option.

1. Cook rice according to package directions.

2. Preheat the oven to 400°F. Spray both a 9-inch pie plate and a large cookie sheet with nonstick cooking spray.

3. In a medium bowl, combine rice, egg whites, and Parmesan cheese. Press rice mixture evenly into the prepared pie plate, and bake for 10 minutes. Set aside.

4. Place zucchini, summer squash, and tomato slices evenly on the prepared cookie sheet.

5. In a small bowl, combine Italian seasoning, garlic salt, and olive oil. Drizzle evenly over vegetables using a pastry brush.

6. Roast vegetables for 18 to 20 minutes or until fork-tender. Remove from the oven.

7. Assemble pie by layering ½ of roasted vegetables over crust, topped with ¼ cup grated cheddar. Add remaining vegetables and cover with remaining ½ cup cheese. Return pie to the oven for 3 minutes or until cheese is melted. Let sit for 5 minutes before cutting into 6 wedges. Enjoy with roasted chicken or grilled fish, or enjoy a larger slice for a lighter-fare meal.

Quinoa with Red Peppers and Pine Nuts

This nutty and fragrant grain-based dish is packed with protein.

1 cup *quinoa*, rinsed and drained

2 cups water

1 TB. olive or vegetable oil

1 TB. butter or trans-fat-free margarine

1 medium red bell pepper, ribs and seeds removed, and cut into strips

1 medium celery stalk, diced

¼ cup pine nuts, toasted

Yield: 6 servings
Prep time: 10 minutes
Cook time: 15 to 20 minutes
Serving size: ½ cup
Each serving has:
186 calories
20 g carbohydrates
9.6 g fat
2.6 g fiber
5 g protein

1. In a medium saucepan over high heat, combine quinoa and water. Bring to boil, reduce heat to low, and cook, covered, for 15 minutes or until liquid is absorbed and quinoa is tender.

2. Meanwhile, in a large skillet over medium heat, combine olive oil, butter, red bell pepper, and celery. Cook, stirring, for about 5 minutes or until vegetables are fork-tender.

3. Add cooked quinoa to the skillet and gently mix. Garnish with pine nuts, and enjoy immediately.

 Wellness Words

Quinoa (pronounced *KEEN-wah*) is a South American grain rich in protein. In fact, 1 cup of quinoa contains 8 grams of protein—the same amount in 1 cup of milk or 1 ounce of meat! Rinsing quinoa first reduces saponins, a soapy-tasting compound naturally found on the grain that can leave a bitter taste.

Quinoa and Millet Sauté

As a nice vegetarian entrée or satisfying side, this dish will likely please even the carnivores in your life!

Yield: 4 servings
Prep time: 10 minutes
Cook time: 25 to 30 minutes
Serving size: 1 cup
Each serving has:
178 calories
28 g carbohydrates
5 g fat
3.4 g fiber
4.5 g protein

½ cup *millet*, rinsed and drained

1 TB. olive or vegetable oil

1 medium red bell pepper, ribs and seeds removed, and diced

2 cups reduced-sodium vegetable broth

¼ cup quinoa, rinsed and drained

½ tsp. onion salt

2 TB. chopped fresh parsley

1. In a large skillet over medium heat, combine millet, olive oil, and red bell pepper. Cook, stirring frequently, for 3 to 5 minutes.

2. Add vegetable broth, and bring to a boil. Reduce heat to low, and simmer, covered, for 5 minutes.

3. Add quinoa to the skillet, cover, and simmer for 15 minutes or until liquid has been absorbed. Season with onion salt, and garnish with parsley.

📖 Wellness Words

Millet is a term for various grass crops whose seeds are harvested for use as food. Just like sunflower seeds, millet is often added to bird food, but you don't have to be a bird to enjoy its nutty flavor!

Quinoa Tabbouleh

Fresh and lemony, this protein-packed dish is terrific with grilled fish.

1 cup quinoa, cooked according to pkg. directions and cooled

3 cups finely chopped fresh parsley

$\frac{1}{2}$ cup finely chopped fresh mint

2 medium tomatoes, finely chopped

4 medium carrots, peeled and finely shredded

1 tsp. garlic powder

$\frac{1}{2}$ tsp. onion salt

$\frac{1}{4}$ cup freshly squeezed lemon juice (2 lemons)

$\frac{1}{4}$ cup olive or vegetable oil

Yield: 7 cups
Prep time: 20 minutes
Serving size: 1 cup
Each serving has:
133 calories
13 g carbohydrates
8 g fat
3 g fiber
2.4 g protein

1. In a large serving bowl, combine quinoa, parsley, mint, to-matoes, and carrots. Set aside.

2. In a small bowl, whisk together garlic powder, onion salt, lemon juice, and olive oil.

3. Drizzle dressing over quinoa mixture, and stir to evenly dis-perse dressing. Store *tabbouleh* in the refrigerator for a great snack served with pitas or the Lemon-Eggplant Dip (recipe in Chapter 13).

 Wellness Words _____

Tabbouleh is a popular Middle Eastern cold salad. In fact, it's my son Kevin's favorite vegetable source! Traditionally made with cracked wheat or bulgur, this recipe substitutes quinoa, the fast-cooking protein-packed grain.

Kasha Pilaf

In this sweet, nutty, and savory dish, you'll enjoy the subtle taste of kasha.

Yield: 7 servings	
Prep time: 10 minutes	
Cook time: 22 minutes	
Serving size: ½ cup	
Each serving has:	
113 calories	
19 g carbohydrates	
3.3 g fat	
3 g fiber	
3 g protein	

1 TB. olive or vegetable oil

2 cloves garlic, cut in half

2 medium celery stalks, finely chopped

2 medium carrots, peeled and finely chopped

1 cup whole kasha (buckwheat groats)

2 cups reduced-sodium low-fat chicken broth

2 TB. almonds, slivered

2 TB. finely chopped fresh parsley

1. In a large saucepan over medium-low heat, combine olive oil and garlic. Cook, stirring frequently, for 1 minute. Using a fork, remove garlic pieces and discard.

2. Stir in celery, carrots, and kasha, and cook for 1 minute. Slowly add chicken broth, and increase heat to medium-high. Bring to a boil, reduce heat to low, and cover. Simmer for 20 minutes.

3. Garnish with almond slivers and parsley, and enjoy immediately.

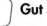

Gut Facts

Kasha is also known as buckwheat groats, but don't be fooled—there's no gluten or wheat in this whole grain. For maximum freshness, store kasha in the refrigerator or freezer. Kasha has a subtle flavor so it easily combines with savory or sweet ingredients.

Seasoned Skillet Millet

This light and nutty side dish will make your taste buds happy.

¾ cup millet, rinsed and drained

2¼ cups water

1 cup grape tomatoes, cut in half

½ tsp. garlic salt

2 TB. finely chopped fresh parsley

Yield: 4 cups
Prep time: 5 minutes
Cook time: 20 minutes
Serving size: 1 cup
Each serving has:
148 calories
28.5 g carbohydrates
1.5 g fat
4 g fiber
5 g protein

1. In a large skillet over medium-high heat, add millet. Cook, stirring frequently, for 30 to 60 seconds or until millet has started to pop and crackle.

2. Slowly add water, and bring to a rolling boil. Reduce heat to low, cover, and cook for 15 to 20 more minutes or until water is absorbed.

3. Add tomatoes, and gently stir. Cook for 1 minute, and remove from heat. Season with garlic salt, garnish with parsley, and serve.

 Digestibles _____

Adding whole grains to your diet is a great way to boost your fiber intake. A high fiber intake may lower your risk of heart disease and colon cancer.

Chapter 21

Cookies and Bars You'll Crave

In This Chapter

- ◆ Chewy and nourishing cookies galore
- ◆ Melt-in-your-mouth brownies and bars
- ◆ Tasty granola bars and other oatmeal goodies

If you're craving a bit of sweets, this chapter gives you a lot to smile about. Unlike commercially made baked goods filled with high-fructose corn syrup and a pile of refined grains, these terrific recipes are concocted with a variety of wholesome grains, fruits, nuts, and nut butters.

Many of the recipes in this chapter have been adapted to contain more heart-friendly oils, instead of the solid fats often found in most cookie and bar recipes, making these treats even healthier for you! Don't be surprised if your belly tolerates these better than your typical favorite sweets, because they've been carefully designed to keep you feeling your best. Just try not to be *too* gluttonous with the sweet stuff, and stick to the serving size!

Oatmeal Cookies

These chewy, nutty oatmeal cookies that take a nutritious turn on Grandma's recipe will be a new family favorite.

Yield: 40 cookies
Prep time: 10 minutes
Cook time: 5 to 7 minutes per batch
Serving size: 2 cookies
Each serving has:
207 calories
26 g carbohydrates
10 g fat
2 g fiber
3 g protein

½ cup butter, at room temperature

½ cup vegetable oil

½ cup brown sugar, firmly packed

½ cup sugar

1 large egg

1 tsp. pure vanilla extract

1½ cups all-purpose flour

1 tsp. baking soda

2½ cups old-fashioned oats

¾ cup *oat flour*

1. Preheat the oven to 350°F. Spray a nonstick cookie sheet with nonstick cooking spray.

2. In a large bowl, combine butter, vegetable oil, brown sugar, and sugar. Mix with a spoon or an electric mixer on medium speed for 2 minutes or until creamy. Stir in egg and vanilla extract.

3. Add flour, baking soda, old-fashioned oats, and oat flour, and mix to blend.

4. Drop dough by the rounded teaspoon onto the prepared cookie sheet about 2 inches apart. Bake for 5 to 7 minutes per batch for a chewy cookie.

Wellness Words

Oat flour consists of whole oats that have been ground to a flour consistency. It's a good source of soluble fiber. Look for it in a health store or in the health section of some grocery stores. If you can't find oat flour, you can create your own by grinding old-fashioned oats in your blender.

Chocolate-Chip Meringues

Light, and with a hint of vanilla, these airy cookies are low in calories and fat. Enjoy one, two, or maybe three!

3 eggs, at room temperature

¼ tsp. cream of tartar

¾ cup superfine sugar

¼ tsp. pure vanilla extract

½ cup mini semisweet chocolate chips

Yield: 26 cookies
Prep time: 15 minutes
Cook time: 2 hours per batch
Serving size: 2 cookies
Each serving has:
80 calories
16 g carbohydrates
1 g fat
0 g fiber
1 g protein

1. Preheat the oven to 300°F.

2. In a small bowl, crack eggs and remove egg yolks, leaving egg whites. (You can do this easily by cracking open the egg over a bowl and allowing the whites to fall into the bowl while moving the yolk from one eggshell half to the other.)

3. Add cream of tartar, and with an electric mixer on medium to high speed, beat mixture for about 2 minutes or until soft peaks form. (The mixture will be able to curl when you pull up the beater.)

4. Slowly add sugar to egg whites ¼ cup at a time along with vanilla extract, and mixture will become even stiffer. Fold in chocolate chips, and drop meringues by the heaping teaspoonful onto a nonstick cookie sheet about 2 inches apart.

5. Place cookie sheet in the oven, and immediately reduce the heat to 200°F. Bake for 2 hours. Remove and cool completely. These cookies are best within the first day of cooking while they're still crispy and light.

Digestibles _____

To make superfine sugar at home, add regular granulated sugar to your food processor fitted with a metal blade, or a blender, and process for 30 seconds. This superfine sugar incorporates easier in recipes like these delicate meringue cookies!

Creamy Peanut Butter Cookies

This is a nutty cookie with a fruity finish! The orange is a nice surprise to your taste buds—and a good way to get some extra vitamin C in your diet.

Yield: 26 cookies
Prep time: 15 minutes
Cook time: 8 to 10 minutes per batch
Serving size: 2 cookies
Each serving has:
259 calories
32 g carbohydrates
12 g fat
2 g fiber
5 g protein

Gut Facts

All-natural peanut butter does not contain hydrogenated fats, the unhealthy fats linked with heart disease risk. Teddie Super Chunky Old Fashioned All Natural Peanut Butter is a great choice for this recipe. Speaking of good brands, King Arthur makes a nice white whole-wheat flour.

$\frac{1}{2}$ **cup butter, at room temperature**

$\frac{1}{2}$ **cup all-natural crunchy peanut butter**

$\frac{1}{2}$ **cup firmly packed brown sugar**

$\frac{3}{4}$ **cup sugar**

1 large egg

3 TB. freshly squeezed orange juice (about 1 orange)

$\frac{1}{2}$ **tsp. orange zest**

$1\frac{3}{4}$ **cups white whole-wheat flour**

$\frac{1}{2}$ **tsp. pure vanilla extract**

1 tsp. baking soda

$\frac{1}{4}$ **tsp. salt**

1. Preheat the oven to 350°F.

2. In a large mixing bowl, combine butter, peanut butter, brown sugar, and $\frac{1}{2}$ cup sugar. Mix with electric mixer on medium speed for 2 minutes or until light and creamy.

3. Beat in egg, orange juice, and orange zest, blending for 1 more minute.

4. Add flour, vanilla extract, baking soda, and salt, and blend for 1 more minute.

5. Scoop out dough by the heaping teaspoon and roll into small balls. Place 2 inches apart on a nonstick cookie sheet, and decorate by making an impression with a fork in a criss-cross pattern. To do this, place remaining $\frac{1}{4}$ cup sugar on a small plate. Dip the fork in sugar in between decorating to ensure the fork doesn't stick to dough.

6. Bake for 8 to 10 minutes or until lightly browned on the edges.

Variation: For **Creamy Chocolate–Peanut Butter Cookies,** add $\frac{1}{2}$ cup mini semisweet chocolate chips to prepared dough and stir by hand until chips are evenly dispersed, about 1 minute.

No-Bake Chocolate Cookies

Chocolate and peanut butter—it's a match made in heaven, and it makes these cookies *so* yummy! *(Adapted and reprinted with permission for IBSFree.net by Patsy Catsos, R.D.)*

½ cup butter or trans-fat-free margarine

2 cups sugar

½ cup reduced-lactose low-fat milk

¾ cup smooth peanut butter

3 cups quick oats

6 TB. cocoa powder

2 tsp. pure vanilla extract

Yield: 24 cookies
Prep time: 35 minutes
Cook time: 2 minutes
Serving size: 1 cookie
Each serving has:
188 calories
25 g carbohydrates
9 g fat
1.8 g fiber
3 g protein

1. In a medium saucepan over medium-high heat, combine butter, sugar, and milk. Bring to a rolling boil, and boil for 1 minute.

2. Add peanut butter, oats, cocoa powder, and vanilla extract, and stir to combine. Remove from heat.

3. Drop by the rounded teaspoonful on a cookie sheet lined with waxed paper. Refrigerate for 30 minutes before serving.

 Gut Facts _____

Quick oats work best in this no-bake recipe because they're rolled thinner than old-fashioned oats and therefore cook quicker. And be sure you use pure vanilla extract in all these other yummy desserts. Pure vanilla extract is derived from the vanilla bean and provides a rich vanilla flavor, while artificial vanilla extract is derived from artificial flavorings.

Lemon Drop Cookies

These cute little drop cookies are just sweet enough with a nice infusion of lemon.

Yield: 24 cookies
Prep time: 20 minutes
Cook time: 10 minutes
Serving size: 2 cookies
Each serving has:
150 calories
22 g carbohydrates
6 g fat
.5 g fiber
1.5 g protein

2 TB. plus ¼ cup sugar

2 TB. butter or trans-fat-free margarine, at room temperature

3 TB. vegetable oil

1 large egg

2 TB. water

½ tsp. lemon extract

1½ cups white rice flour

1 tsp. baking soda

2 TB. freshly squeezed lemon juice (1 lemon)

1. Preheat the oven to 350°F. Spray a nonstick cookie sheet with nonstick cooking spray.

2. In a medium bowl, blend 2 tablespoons sugar, butter, and vegetable oil with a spoon until creamy. Mix in egg, water, and lemon extract.

3. Add flour, baking soda, and lemon juice, and stir until well blended.

4. Pour remaining ¼ cup sugar on a small plate.

5. Form small balls of dough about 1½ inch in diameter, and dip one side of ball in sugar. Place on the prepared cookie sheet, sugar side up, about 2 inches apart. Bake for 10 minutes. These cookies are best warm from the oven.

Gut Facts

Rice flour is wheat- and gluten-free, making it a nice alternative for wheat-sensitive folks. Find white rice flour in health food stores or possibly in the gluten-free section of your local grocery store.

Cornmeal-Cranberry Biscotti

Fruity and light, these crunchy cookies pair nicely with a warm cup of tea.

½ cup all-purpose flour

½ cup white whole-wheat flour

½ cup finely ground cornmeal

½ tsp. baking powder

4 TB. butter, at room temperature

3 TB. vegetable oil

½ cup sugar

½ tsp. pure vanilla extract

1 large egg

1 tsp. orange zest

¼ cup dried cranberries, chopped

3 TB. white chocolate chips

Yield: 18 biscotti
Prep time: 15 to 20 minutes
Cook time: 10 to 12 minutes
Serving size: 1 biscotti
Each serving has:
121 calories
15 g carbohydrates
5.8 g fat
1 g fiber
1.3 g protein

1. In a small mixing bowl, combine all-purpose flour, white whole-wheat flour, cornmeal, and baking powder. Set aside.

2. In a medium bowl, combine butter, vegetable oil, sugar, vanilla extract, egg, and orange zest. With electric mixer on medium speed, blend well, slowly adding cornmeal mixture. It will be a crumbly mixture.

3. Add cranberries, and mix with a spoon until well dispersed throughout dough.

4. On a large piece of parchment paper, form dough into an 8×4-inch rectangle about ¾ inch high. Cover with another sheet of parchment paper, and refrigerate for 2 hours to firm dough.

5. Preheat the oven to 350°F. Spray a nonstick cookie sheet with nonstick cooking spray.

6. Remove dough from the refrigerator, and cut into strips about ¾ inch thick. Place strips on the prepared cookie sheet, and bake for 10 to 12 minutes or until lightly browned.

7. Place white chocolate chips in a small, microwave-safe dish. Microwave for 10 seconds on high power, and stir with a fork to blend. To decorate cookies, get some chocolate on the fork, hold it above the biscotti, and drizzle the melted chocolate over the cookies.

Gut Facts

Cornmeal is a good source of phosphorus and magnesium. Both of these nutrients help keep your bones healthy!

Crispy Rice Treats

Fiber-rich cereal gives this old-fashioned favorite a healthful kick!

Yield: 20 squares
Prep time: 5 minutes
Cook time: 5 to 10 minutes
Serving size: 1 square
Each serving has:
92 calories
21 g carbohydrates
2.6 g fat
1.8 g fiber
1 g protein

3 cups crisp rice cereal

3 cups Barbara's Bakery Ultima Organic High Fiber cereal

2 TB. vegetable oil

2 TB. butter or trans-fat-free margarine

1 (10.5-oz.) pkg. mini marshmallows

1. In a large bowl, combine crispy rice cereal and Barbara's Bakery Ultima Organic High Fiber cereal.

2. In a large stockpot over medium heat, combine vegetable oil, butter, and marshmallows, stirring constantly.

3. When marshmallows have all melted, add cereal mixture to marshmallows, and remove the pot from heat. Thoroughly blend cereal and marshmallow mixture.

4. Spray a 9×13-inch pan with nonstick cooking spray.

5. Transfer rice mixture to the prepared 9×13 pan, pressing firmly into an even layer. Let sit for 15 minutes before cutting into 20 squares.

 Digestibles

Barbara's Bakery has a fine selection of whole-grain cereals. You can find them at many major grocery chains.

Brownie Bites

If you're looking for rich and chocolaty, you've come to the right place—and they're both in one bite-size brownie!

4 extra-large eggs

1½ cups sugar

4 TB. butter or trans-fat-free margarine, melted and cooled

¼ cup vegetable oil

2 tsp. pure vanilla extract

½ cup all-purpose flour

1¼ cups cocoa powder, sifted

¼ cup prune purée

2 TB. confectioners' sugar

Yield: 48 mini brownies
Prep time: 15 minutes
Cook time: 15 to 20 minutes
Serving size: 2 brownies
Each serving has:
126 calories
19 g carbohydrates
5 g fat
1 g fiber
2 g protein

1. Preheat the oven to 350°F. Spray one or more nonstick mini muffin tins, enough for 48 brownies, with nonstick cooking spray.

2. In a large bowl, combine eggs and sugar. Add butter, vegetable oil, and vanilla extract, and mix well with a spoon. Add flour, cocoa powder, and prune purée, and mix well.

3. Add brownie mixture to the prepared muffin tin by the teaspoon, filling ¾ full. Bake for 15 to 20 minutes or until a cake tester inserted into the center comes out clean.

4. Remove brownies from the oven, let cool, and run a butter knife around the edge of the tin to help loosen. Remove brownies, and place on a plate.

5. Place confectioners' sugar in a sieve or a sifter, and sprinkle over top of brownies.

Digestibles

You can make prune purée and keep it in the refrigerator for 3 or 4 days. For 1 cup purée, combine 1⅓ cups pitted prunes and 6 tablespoons water in a food processor fitted with a metal blade. Pulse on and off until prunes are finely chopped. For just enough for this recipe, blend 6 prunes with 2 tablespoons water. You can use prune purée as a fat substitute in hearty muffin or cookie recipes. Simply substitute half the fat with an equal amount of prune purée. Prunes are a good source of fiber and FODMAPs—and help eliminate constipation issues!

Oat 'n' Cranberry Squares

These sandwiched layers of sweet oats are reminiscent of raspberry squares but with a twist of orange and cranberry filling.

Yield: 12 squares
Prep time: 15 minutes
Cook time: 35 minutes
Serving size: 1 square
Each serving has:
167 calories
22 g carbohydrates
8 g fat
2 g fiber
2 g protein

1 cup fresh cranberries

1 orange, washed, peeled, and ½ of peel reserved

2 TB. plus ¼ cup sugar

1½ TB. cornstarch

½ cup butter, cold, cut into pieces

¼ cup firmly packed brown sugar

½ tsp. ground cinnamon

1 cup all-purpose flour

1 cup old-fashioned oats

2 TB. confectioners' sugar (optional)

Digestibles

You can use the cranberry-orange mixture straight from the food processor as a great relish alongside grilled fish or a roasted chicken dinner. Yum!

1. Preheat the oven to 350°F. Spray an 8-inch-square pan with nonstick cooking spray.

2. In a food processor fitted with a metal blade, combine cranberries, peeled orange, ½ of orange peel, and 2 tablespoons sugar. Pulse for 2 minutes or until finely ground.

3. In a small saucepan over medium heat, add cranberry mixture and cornstarch, stirring constantly for 5 minutes until thickened like a hearty jam. Set aside.

4. In a medium bowl, combine butter, brown sugar, remaining ¼ cup sugar, cinnamon, flour, and oats. Mix using a pastry blender or 2 forks until mixture resembles fine crumbs.

5. In the prepared 8-inch-square pan, sprinkle ½ of oat mixture, and press firmly in the pan. Bake for 10 minutes.

6. Remove the pan from the oven, and spread cranberry-orange mixture evenly over oat crust, crumble remaining oat mixture on top, and bake for 25 more minutes.

7. Remove from the oven, let sit for 20 minutes, and cut into 12 squares. Sprinkle with confectioners' sugar (if using).

Granola Bars

These hearty, nutty granola bars will stick to your ribs! Enjoy these bars as a great snack on the go.

½ cup oat bran

2 cups quick oats

3 TB. ground flaxseed or flaxseed meal

½ cup dried cranberries, finely chopped

⅔ cup unsalted roasted almonds, finely chopped

¼ cup unsalted sunflower seeds

¼ cup maple syrup

2 TB. firmly packed brown sugar

⅓ cup almond nut butter

1 tsp. pure vanilla extract

¼ cup vegetable oil

Yield: 15 bars
Prep time: 10 minutes, plus 3 or 4 hours refrigerate time
Cook time: 2 or 3 minutes
Serving size: 1 bar
Each serving has:
192 calories
21 g carbohydrates
11 g fat
3 g fiber
4 g protein

1. In a large bowl, combine oat bran, oats, flaxseed, cranberries, almonds, and sunflower seeds. Set aside.

2. In a small saucepan over medium heat, combine maple syrup, brown sugar, almond nut butter, vanilla extract, and vegetable oil.. Cook, stirring constantly, for 2 minutes or until mixture is creamy. Remove from heat.

3. Spray an 8-inch nonstick baking pan with nonstick cooking spray.

4. Pour nut butter mixture into oat mixture, and mix well. Press mixture firmly into the prepared 8-inch nonstick baking pan. Refrigerate for 3 or 4 hours to firm granola bars.

5. Using a sharp knife, cut into 15 pieces. Store individually in snack-size zipper-lock bags for an easy grab-and-go snack. These will last in the refrigerator for up to 3 or 4 days.

Gut Facts

Flaxseed is a great source of soluble fiber and a plant source of omega-3 fats, both of which are your heart's friends. Before your body can digest the flaxseed, it needs to be ground, so look for flaxseed meal in the natural section of your grocery store or grind your own in a coffee mill or food processor. Refrigerate flaxseed because it can become rancid more quickly at room temperature.

Chapter 22

Delectable Cakes, Tarts, and Other Sweet Treats

In This Chapter

- ◆ Fruit- and veggie-filled cakes and treats
- ◆ Flourless creations
- ◆ Chocolate delicacies
- ◆ Frozen concoctions

This book wouldn't be complete without a chapter or two dedicated to sweet treats! In this chapter, you will find lots of great desserts that just happen to have a few nutritional extras, too, so feel free to enjoy these guilt-free goodies when it's time to indulge your sweet tooth.

There's nothing better than nature's gift of fresh, mouthwatering fruit to give your body its dose of needed daily vitamins and minerals. Vibrant-colored fruits and vegetables also provide key phytochemicals. These important plant substances are linked with lowering risk of chronic diseases such as cancer and heart disease. Rest assured, many of the recipes in this chapter sneak in some of Mother Nature's wholesome foods in almost every sweet little bite.

Banana Cake

A great way to use over-ripe bananas, this cake is divinely dense and fruity with a big hint of cinnamon.

Yield: 16 servings
Prep time: 10 minutes
Cook time: 30 to 35 minutes
Serving size: 1 square
Each serving has:
168 calories
24 g carbohydrates
7.5 g fat
1 g fiber
2 g protein

½ cup vegetable oil

3 large ripe bananas, peeled and mashed

¾ cup sugar

2 large eggs

1¼ cups all-purpose flour

1 tsp. baking soda

1 TB. ground cinnamon

2 TB. confectioners' sugar

1. Preheat the oven to 350°F. Spray an 8-inch-square nonstick pan with nonstick cooking spray.

2. In a medium bowl, combine vegetable oil, bananas, and sugar. Blend with a spoon to mix. Add eggs, and stir.

3. Sift flour, baking soda, and cinnamon. Add to egg mixture, and blend.

4. Pour into the prepared 8-inch-square pan, and bake for 20 minutes. After 20 minutes, cover the pan with aluminum foil to keep cake from overbrowning, and cook 10 to 15 more minutes or until a cake tester inserted into the center comes out clean.

5. Sift confectioner's sugar over top of cake, and enjoy.

 Gut Facts

Bananas are a great source of potassium, but did you know they are a great source of fiber and a good source of vitamin C, too?

Pumpkin Cake

When the weather turns cool, this spicy cake with creamy filling is a seasonal favorite!

⅔ cup canned pumpkin

3 large eggs

½ cup sugar

¾ cup all-purpose flour

1 tsp. baking soda

½ tsp. ground cinnamon

1½ tsp. pure vanilla extract

1 (8-oz.) pkg. reduced-fat cream cheese or *Neufchâtel cheese*, at room temperature

1 TB. butter, at room temperature

1 cup confectioners' sugar

Yield: 10 pieces
Prep time: 15 to 20 minutes
Cook time: 15 to 20 minutes
Serving size: 1 round slice, about ¹⁄₁₀ cake
Each serving has:
214 calories
31 g carbohydrates
8 g fat
1 g fiber
5 g protein

1. Preheat the oven to 350°F. Line an 11×15-inch jelly-roll pan with parchment paper.

2. In a large mixing bowl, combine pumpkin, eggs, and sugar mixing with electric mixer on medium speed for 1 or 2 minutes. Add flour, baking soda, cinnamon, and ½ teaspoon vanilla extract, and blend for 1 or 2 more minutes.

3. Pour pumpkin mixture on the prepared jelly-roll pan, and spread out in an even rectangular layer about ¼ to ½ inch thick. (This might not cover the entire pan.)

4. Bake for 15 to 20 minutes or until a cake tester inserted into the center comes out clean. Remove from oven and let cool.

5. In a medium bowl, combine cream cheese, butter, confectioners' sugar, and remaining 1 teaspoon vanilla extract. Beat mixture with electric mixer on medium speed for 2 or 3 minutes or until well blended and creamy.

6. Spread frosting on cooled cake, and roll into a jelly-roll shape, starting with short end of cake. Refrigerate log, letting icing set for 1 hour. Using a sharp knife, cut into 1-inch pieces. Serve cake on its side, exposing the pinwheel pattern.

Wellness Words

Neufchâtel **cheese** is a soft, unripened cheese originating from France. It's often used as a low-fat variety of cream cheese. Its wonderful flavor complements the pumpkin in this cake.

Strawberry Shortcake

This summer dessert is great when fresh strawberries are at their finest.

Yield: 8 servings
Prep time: 20 minutes
Cook time: 8 to 10 minutes
Serving size: 1 shortcake and ¾ cup berries
Each serving has:
279 calories
35 g carbohydrates
12 g fat
3 g fiber
5.5 g protein

2 cups plus 2 TB. white whole-wheat flour

1½ TB. baking powder

4 TB. plus 2 tsp. sugar

½ cup butter, chilled and chopped small

⅔ cup reduced-lactose low-fat milk

6 cups strawberries, hulled and chopped (about 2 lb.)

2 TB. freshly squeezed lemon juice (1 lemon)

1 (14-oz.) can whipped cream (optional)

1. Preheat the oven to 350°F. Spray a nonstick cookie sheet with nonstick cooking spray.

2. In a large bowl, combine 2 cups flour, baking powder, 4 tablespoons sugar, and butter. Mix with a pastry blender or 2 forks until mixture resembles crumbs. Make a well in center of crumb mixture, and slowly incorporate milk with a fork. Don't overmix. Let sit a minute or two.

3. On a clean countertop or a large piece of wax paper, sprinkle remaining 2 tablespoons flour, and add dough. Knead dough by pushing down and flipping it to get a smooth consistency. Divide dough into 8 equal pieces, and lightly roll into balls.

4. Place rolled dough onto the prepared cookie sheet. Sprinkle evenly with 1 teaspoon sugar, and bake for 8 to 10 minutes. Remove and let sit for 5 minutes.

5. Meanwhile, in a large bowl, gently combine strawberries, lemon juice, and remaining 1 teaspoon sugar.

6. Top a warm biscuit with ¾ cup strawberries, and garnish with 1 tablespoon whipped cream (if using).

Variation: If strawberries aren't in season or you prefer another fruit, you can substitute blueberries, raspberries, or a mixture of your favorite berries instead.

Gut Facts

The white whole-wheat flour in this recipe has all the fiber, vitamins, and minerals of traditional whole-wheat flour, but it's made from a white variety of wheat. That gives it a lighter color and texture in baked goods.

Mini Chocolate Pudding Tarts

These creamy, easy-to-make tarts are a fan favorite at football parties or make a kid-friendly afternoon snack!

¾ cup graham cracker crumbs

3 TB. butter or trans-fat-free margarine, melted

1 tsp. plus ½ cup sugar

⅓ cup cocoa powder, sifted

3 TB. cornstarch

2 cups reduced-lactose low-fat milk

2 tsp. pure vanilla extract

Yield: 48 mini tarts
Prep time: 10 minutes plus 1 hour refrigerate time
Cook time: 5 minutes
Serving size: 2 tarts
Each serving has:
59 calories
9 g carbohydrates
2 g fat
0 g fiber
1 g protein

1. Line one or more nonstick mini muffin tins, enough for 48 tarts, with paper liners.

2. In a medium bowl, combine graham cracker crumbs, butter, and 1 teaspoon sugar, and mix with a fork.

3. Add 1 heaping teaspoon crumb mixture to each lined muffin tin, filling about ⅓ full. Press mixture firmly into each liner. Set aside.

4. In a microwave-safe dish, combine remaining ½ cup sugar with cocoa powder and cornstarch. With a fork, slowly add milk and vanilla extract to reach a smooth consistency. Dry ingredients will want to float on top of milk, so push them down with the fork while blending.

5. Microwave on high power for 2 minutes. Remove and stir well to ensure even cooking. Return to microwave and cook for 1 more minute. Remove, stir, and continue this process for 1 or 2 more minutes or until pudding is thick.

6. Add 1 heaping teaspoon thickened pudding on top of each graham cracker crust, filling ¾ full. Cover muffin tin with plastic wrap, and refrigerate for about 1 hour or until set.

🗨 Gut Facts

Milk-rich pudding can be problematic for the lactose-intolerant IBS sufferer, but these bite-size pudding tarts made with reduced-lactose milk have just a trace of lactose, so enjoy without worry!

Berry Crisp

Sweet and tangy berries combine beautifully with the crunchy whole-grain topping in this lovely crisp.

Yield: 6 servings
Prep time: 10 minutes
Cook time: 1 hour
Serving size: ⅙ pan
Each serving has:
392 calories
62 g carbohydrates
14 g fat
5 g fiber
4 g protein

2 (16-oz.) bags frozen mixed berries

1 TB. plus ¼ cup sugar

1 cup all-purpose flour

1 TB. lemon juice

¾ cup old-fashioned oats

⅔ cup firmly packed brown sugar

1 tsp. ground cinnamon

½ tsp. ground ginger

7 TB. butter, chilled and chopped small

1. Preheat the oven to 350°F. Spray an 8-inch-square baking dish with nonstick cooking spray.

2. In a medium bowl, combine frozen berries with 1 tablespoon sugar, ¼ cup flour, and lemon juice. Transfer berries to the prepared dish.

3. In a medium bowl, combine remaining ¾ cup flour, oats, brown sugar, cinnamon, and ginger. Add butter, and using a pastry blender or 2 forks, blend butter into flour mixture until it resembles crumbs. Sprinkle over berries.

4. Bake for 1 hour or until bubbling. Let sit for 15 minutes prior to serving.

Digestibles _____

There's no need to defrost the berries for this recipe, so it's a great quick-fix dessert. You can even make the topping earlier in the day, or the day before, for a speedy last-minute assembly. Pop the dessert in the oven right as you sit down to eat, and this wholesome fruit crisp will be ready when you're all set for dessert.

Fresh Fruit Salad with Mint

All ages will enjoy this refreshing and light dessert.

1 banana, peeled and cut into thin rounds

1 cup fresh strawberries, hulled and cut in half

1 cup fresh blackberries

1 cup fresh blueberries

1 TB. lemon juice

1 TB. sugar

2 TB. chopped fresh mint

Yield: *4 servings*		
Prep time: 10 minutes		
Serving size: 1 cup		
Each serving has:		
95 calories		
23 g carbohydrates		
0 g fat		
5 g fiber		
1 g protein		

1. In a medium serving bowl, combine banana, strawberries, blackberries, blueberries, lemon juice, and sugar.

2. Garnish with fresh mint, and serve immediately.

 Gut Facts

Fruit salad is a great sweet snack packed with loads of vitamins and minerals.

Creamy Quinoa Pudding

Talk about comfort foods! This creamy cinnamon and vanilla–infused pudding makes the top of my list!

Yield: 6 servings
Prep time: 5 minutes plus 2 hours chill time
Cook time: 20 to 23 minutes
Serving size: ½ cup
Each serving has:
168 calories
23 g carbohydrates
4.5 g fat
1 g fiber
8 g protein

½ cup quinoa, rinsed and drained

3 cups reduced-lactose low-fat milk

2 large eggs

¼ cup sugar

¼ tsp. ground cinnamon

1 tsp. pure vanilla extract

1. In a large saucepan over medium-high heat, add quinoa and milk. Bring to a boil, reduce heat to low, and simmer, stirring occasionally, for about 15 minutes or until soft.

2. In a small mixing bowl, whisk together eggs, sugar, cinnamon, and vanilla extract.

3. Slowly add egg mixture to quinoa while stirring. Cook for 5 to 8 more minutes or until thickened.

4. Pour ½ cup pudding into 6 (6-ounce) serving dishes, cover with plastic wrap, and refrigerate for at least 2 hours prior to eating.

 Gut Facts

This pudding is jam-packed with protein, thanks to the quinoa and milk!

Flourless Chocolate Torte

This dessert is about as rich as it gets, and a small sliver will meet the expectation of all chocoholics!

2 cups semisweet chocolate chips

9 TB. butter

4 large eggs

½ cup sugar

1 tsp. pure vanilla extract

1 TB. confectioners' sugar (optional)

1 cup fresh raspberries (optional)

Yield: 16 servings
Prep time: 5 to 10 minutes
Cook time: 25 minutes
Serving size: $\frac{1}{16}$ torte
Each serving has:
141 calories
11.6 g carbohydrates
10 g fat
0 g fiber
1.5 g protein

1. Preheat the oven to 325°F. Spray a 9-inch springform pan with nonstick cooking spray.

2. Place chocolate chips and butter in a microwave-safe dish. Microwave on high power for 30 seconds. Remove from microwave, stir, and microwave for 30 more seconds. Repeat cooking for 30 seconds and stirring until chocolate and butter are melted and creamy. Be careful not to burn chocolate. Set aside.

3. In a medium bowl, beat eggs with an electric mixer on medium-high speed for about 2 or 3 minutes or until pale and double in size. Gradually add sugar and vanilla extract. Slowly add chocolate mixture, ¼ cup at a time, until all chocolate has been added.

4. Pour chocolate mixture into the prepared springform pan. Bake on the middle oven rack for 25 minutes. Remove from the oven, and let sit for 10 minutes.

5. Run a butter knife around the edges of the pan before opening the spring closure. Sprinkle confectioners' sugar (if using) over top of tort, and top with fresh raspberries (if using).

 Gut Facts

Made without any wheat, rye, or barley flour, this torte is safe for those on a gluten-free diet.

Angel Food Cake with Berries

The vanilla cake complements the sweet and lemony berry mixture. Add this dessert to your repertoire, and it will make your busy weeknight routine a little more special.

Yield: 12 servings
Prep time: 5 minutes plus 2 hours defrost time
Serving size: $\frac{1}{12}$ cake with 2 tablespoons fruit mixture
Each serving has:
89 calories
20 g carbohydrates
0 g fat
1 g fiber
1.6 g protein

1 (16-oz.) pkg. frozen mixed berries, defrosted in the refrigerator for 2 hours, and drained

2 TB. freshly squeezed lemon juice (1 lemon)

1 TB. Grand Marnier

1 tsp. sugar

1 store-bought angel food cake

1. In a medium bowl, combine mixed berries, lemon juice, Grand Marnier, and sugar.

2. Slice angel food cake into 12 slices. Drizzle each slice with 2 tablespoons berry mixture, and serve.

Digestibles

Kick up this recipe a notch by adding 1 tablespoon lemon sorbet on top. If you'd prefer not to add the Grand Marnier, which is an orange-flavored liqueur, simply add 1 teaspoon orange zest instead for flavor.

Orange Zest Sorbet

What a refreshing treat on a hot summer day!

1¼ cups water

⅓ cup sugar

1 cup freshly squeezed orange juice, with pulp (2 medium oranges)

1 TB. orange zest

Yield: *3 servings*
Prep time: 5 minutes plus 2 hours freeze time
Cook time: 1 minute
Serving size: ½ cup
Each serving has:
96 calories
22 g carbohydrates
0 g fat
0 g fiber
.6 g protein

1. In a small saucepan over high heat, combine water and sugar. Stir for 1 minute or until sugar is completely dissolved. Remove the pan from heat, and let mixture cool for 10 minutes.

2. Combine cooled sugar mixture with orange juice and orange zest. Pour mixture into a plastic bowl, cover with plastic wrap, and freeze for a minimum of 2 hours. Scoop out and enjoy!

Gut Facts

The orange juice in this chilled dessert gives you a big dose of vitamin C. Vitamin C is a powerful antioxidant, with disease-fighting properties.

Brennan's Homemade Frozen Lemonade

You'll love this refreshingly sweet and tart slushy.

Yield: 3 cups
Prep time: 5 minutes
Serving size: 1 cup
Each serving has:
71 calories
18 g carbohydrates
0 g fat
0 g fiber
0 g protein

3 cups ice

$\frac{1}{3}$ cup freshly squeezed lemon juice (2 lemons)

$\frac{1}{4}$ cup sugar

1 cup water

1. In a blender, combine ice, lemon juice, sugar, and water.

2. Blend for 1 or 2 minutes or until smooth and slushy. Serve in a wine glass.

Gut Facts

Lemons are a great source of vitamin C. They're also highly acidic, which is why they make your mouth pucker when you eat them!

Grapefruit Granita

This sweet and tangy ice-filled treat is a nice finish to a rich meal.

1 cup grapefruit juice

2 cups water

¼ cup sugar

½ cup fresh blueberries (optional)

Fresh mint leaves

Yield: 3 cups
Prep time: 1½ to 2 hours
Serving size: 1 cup
Each serving has:
96 calories
24 g carbohydrates
0 g fat
0 g fiber
0 g protein

1. In a medium saucepan over high heat, combine grapefruit juice, water, and sugar. Bring to a boil, and cook for 1 or 2 minutes or until sugar is dissolved.

2. Transfer mixture to an 8-inch-square pan, and place in freezer. Every 30 minutes, scrape granita with a fork.

3. Continue to freeze and scrape for about 1½ hours or until granita is completely full of ice crystals and no liquid remains.

4. Serve shaved ice in champagne glasses garnished with fresh blueberries (if using) and fresh mint leaves.

Gut Facts

Grapefruit comes in many varieties, ranging from white, to pink, to red. Try different varieties for this recipe. Ruby red is my favorite. If you're using freshly squeezed grapefruit juice, you'll need 1 large grapefruit for this recipe.

Appendix A

Glossary

alcohol by volume (ABV)   A measurement of the amount of alcohol by volume in an alcoholic beverage.

allergen   A molecule your body recognizes as foreign or dangerous.

amylase   A digestive enzyme that helps digest carbohydrates.

anaphylactic shock   A life-threatening reaction that can cause low blood pressure, labored breathing, swelling of the tongue, and potential heart failure in someone with a true food allergy.

anthocyanins   Plant substances that give plants red, purple, or blue color and are known to have antioxidant properties.

antibodies   Proteins produced by the body in response to what it perceives as intruders or foreign substances.

antioxidants   Substances that prevent oxidative damage to the body. They're linked with decreasing the risk of several kinds of disease.

arborio   A rice that's the key ingredient in making classic Italian risotto. This high-starch, short-grained rice makes a creamy dish.

arugula   A fragrant and peppery green leafy vegetable popular in Italian cuisine.

autoimmune disease   A disease that occurs when your immune system is over-reactive and your body actually attacks itself.

bake   To cook in a dry oven. Dry-heat cooking often results in a crisping of the exterior of the food being cooked. Moist-heat cooking, through methods such as steaming, poaching, etc., brings a much different, moist quality to the food.

basil   A flavorful, almost sweet, resinous herb delicious with tomatoes and used in all kinds of Italian or Mediterranean-style dishes.

beat   To quickly mix substances.

Bibb lettuce   A member of the butter head lettuce family that contains potassium and vitamin A.

bifodobacteria   A healthy bacteria, or probiotic, found in the large intestine.

black pepper   A biting and pungent seasoning, freshly ground pepper is a must for many dishes and adds an extra level of flavor and taste.

blend   To completely mix something, usually with a blender or food processor, more slowly than beating.

boil   To heat a liquid to a point where water is forced to turn into steam, causing the liquid to bubble. To boil something is to insert it into boiling water. A rapid boil is when a lot of bubbles form on the surface of the liquid.

bok choy   A member of the brassica family alongside broccoli and kale. It's a good source of calcium.

breadcrumbs   Tiny pieces of crumbled dry bread. Breadcrumbs are an important component in many recipes and are also used as a coating, for example with breaded chicken breasts.

broth   *See* stock.

brown   To cook in a skillet, turning, until the food's surface is seared and brown in color to lock in the juices.

brown rice   Whole-grain rice including the germ with a characteristic pale brown or tan color. It's more nutritious and flavorful than white rice.

caffeine   A bitter substance found in coffee, tea, and other foods that acts as a stimulant in the body.

capers   Pickled flower buds that offer a tangy flavor to a dish, especially popular in Mediterranean fare. Find brined capers in the pickle and olive section of most grocery stores.

carotenoids   Carotenoids are pigments that provide color to plants. They are believed to help maintain eye health and minimize cancer risk when consumed from deep green, yellow, orange, and red plant foods. The most widely studied carotenoid is beta-carotene.

cayenne   A fiery spice made from (hot) chile peppers, especially the cayenne chile, a slender, red, and very hot pepper.

celiac disease (CD)   An autoimmune disease in which gluten is toxic to the small intestine, causing damage to it.

cheddar   The ubiquitous hard cow's milk cheese with a rich, buttery flavor that ranges from mellow to sharp. Originally produced in England, cheddar is now produced worldwide.

chop   To cut into pieces, usually qualified by an adverb such as "*coarsely* chopped," or by a size measurement such as "chopped into $\frac{1}{2}$-inch pieces." "Finely chopped" is much closer to mince.

chop suey   An American- and Chinese-influenced dish made typically with vegetables, especially bean sprouts, and bite-size meats in a savory, Asian-style sauce.

cilantro   A member of the parsley family used in Mexican cooking and some Asian dishes. Cilantro is what gives some salsas their unique flavor. Use in moderation, as the flavor can overwhelm. The seed of the cilantro is the spice coriander.

cinnamon   A sweet, rich, aromatic spice commonly used in baking or desserts. Cinnamon can also be used for delicious and interesting entrées.

cirrhosis   A scarring of liver tissue as a consequence of liver disease.

coconut cream   A thick liquid made from fresh coconuts, which contains excess fructose.

coconut milk   A product similar to coconut cream but with a greater water content.

complex carbohydrates   Substances that contain multiple chains of sugar molecules often referred to as "starchy" foods.

constipation   An inability to move the bowels on a regular basis, resulting in stool that becomes hard and difficult to pass.

curry   A general term referring to rich, spicy, Indian-style sauces and the dishes prepared with them. A curry will use curry powder as its base seasoning.

devein   The removal of the dark vein from the back of a large shrimp with a sharp knife.

diamine oxidase   The enzyme necessary to break down histamine in the body.

digestive enzymes   Substances released in the digestive tract to aid digestion.

Dijon mustard   A hearty, spicy mustard made in the style of the Dijon region of France.

disaccharides   Carbohydrates that consist of two sugar molecules.

drizzle   To lightly sprinkle drops of a liquid over food. Drizzling is often the finishing touch to a dish.

essential fats   Fats that are obtained from the diet because your body cannot make them on its own.

fat-soluble vitamins   Vitamins that can be dissolved in fat. The fat-soluble vitamins A, D, E, and K are stored in your body's fat or liver.

fermentable carbohydrates (also **fermentable sugars**)   Dietary sugars that are not fully digested and absorbed by the body.

fillet   A piece of meat or seafood with the bones removed.

flaxseed   A seed that's a great source of soluble fiber and a plant source of omega-3 fats.

floret   The flower or bud end of broccoli or cauliflower.

flour   Grains ground into a meal. Wheat is perhaps the most common flour. Flour is also made from oats, rye, buckwheat, soybeans, etc.

FODMAPs   An acronym for the fermentable carbohydrates, known as fermentable oligosaccharides, disaccharides, monosaccharides, and polyols.

food allergy   The reaction of your body's immune system to a food, recognizing the food as foreign. The most common food allergies are wheat, eggs, milk, peanuts, tree nuts, soy, shellfish, and corn.

food diary   A record-keeping journal that details all the foods, beverages, and symptoms associated with consumption.

food intolerance   A negative reaction to food that does not involve the immune system but often does involve the digestive system, such as lactose intolerance.

food sensitivity   A reaction that occurs when your body responds adversely to food. Some food sensitivities cause migraine headaches or eczema, a dry, itchy skin rash.

forbidden rice   A medium Chinese black nutty rice.

frittata   A baked egg dish made of cheese, eggs, meats, and vegetables.

fructans   A type of oligosaccharide comprised of chains of fructose.

fructooligosaccharides (FOS)   Sometimes referred to as oligofructose or oligofructans, FOSes are similar in structure to inulin but typically contain a smaller chain of fructose molecules.

fructose   A simple sugar found in honey and fruits. Excess fructose can be problematic for some people with IBS.

fructose malabsorption   When excess fructose is not digested and causes diarrhea and bloating.

galactans   Oligosaccharides that are comprised on chains of the sugar galactose.

galactose   A simple sugar that, when combined with glucose, makes lactose, the sugar found in milk.

garlic   A member of the onion family, a pungent and flavorful element in many savory dishes. A garlic bulb, the form in which garlic is often sold, contains multiple cloves. Each clove, when chopped, provides about 1 teaspoon garlic. Garlic is rich in fructans and, therefore, can be problematic for those with IBS. Most IBS recipes call for cloves so they can be easily removed prior to eating.

garnish   An embellishment not vital to the dish but added to enhance visual appeal.

gastrocolic reflex   A reflex that triggers intestinal movement or motility with the onset of eating.

ginger   Available in fresh root or dried, ground form, ginger adds a pungent, sweet, and spicy quality to a dish. It's a very popular element of many Asian and Indian dishes, among others.

glucose   One of the simple forms of sugar, also known as monounsaccharides.

gluten   The general name for the storage proteins found in wheat, rye, and barley.

gluten intolerance or sensitivity   The negative reaction your body has to gluten in the diet.

grate   To shave into tiny pieces using a sharp rasp or grater.

Greek yogurt   A type of yogurt that has a creamier consistency than typical yogurts due to the lengthier straining process that removes more of the liquid content. The protein content is also considerably higher.

high-fructose corn syrup (HFCS)   A commonly used sweetener in cookies, crackers, breads, and soda. It can contribute to excess fructose in the diet.

histamine   A protein found in a variety of foods such as beer, pizza, and wine.

histamine intolerance   An inability to break down the histamine found in many foods due to inadequate amounts of the enzyme diamine oxidase (DAO).

honey   A sweet, golden liquid made by insects using nectar from flowers. Honey is rich in excess fructose.

hydrogen or methane breath tests   Testing used to determine small intestinal bacterial overgrowth, lactose intolerance, and fructose malabsorption.

hydrogenated fats   Fats created when liquid oils are converted to solid form. These unhealthy fats are linked to increased risk of heart disease.

insoluble fiber   The fiber found primarily in wheat and vegetables that adds bulk to the stool.

intestinal flora   Bacteria that normally reside in your intestines.

inulin   A plant's storage form of carbohydrates that is widely found in nature. Inulin is made up of long chains of the molecule fructose. Common sources of inulin include wheat, onions, asparagus, garlic, and chicory root.

irritable bowel syndrome (IBS)   A collection of symptoms that occurs in your digestive tract when nerves and muscles do not work correctly. Infections may contribute to this disorder, but in most cases the cause is unknown.

isomalt   A sugar-free sweetener. A source of polyols in the diet.

Italian seasoning (also **spaghetti sauce seasoning**)   The ubiquitous grocery store blend of dried herbs—basil, oregano, rosemary, and thyme. Italian seasoning is a useful blend for quick flavor that evokes the "old country" in sauces, meatballs, soups, and vegetable dishes.

kasha   A whole grain, also known as buckwheat groats, that contains no gluten or wheat.

kefir   A fermented milk drink similar to a drinkable yogurt that may or may not have fruit added to it. Kefir is found in health food stores and is available in plain or fruity varieties.

lactase   The enzyme responsible for breaking down lactose in the body.

lactobacillus   A category of bacteria considered beneficial to the human body.

lactose   The sugar found in milk and many dairy products.

lactose intolerance   The inability to digest the milk sugar lactose due to the lack of lactase production.

lemongrass   A long, yellow, stalklike vegetable commonly used in Asian dishes. You can find it in Asian markets or health food stores.

lycopene   A phytochemical (plant chemical) found in red-colored plant foods. It's linked with lowering the risk of prostate, lung, and stomach cancer and may even lower the risk of heart disease.

malabsorption   When your body has difficulty absorbing nutrients from food.

maltitol   A sugar alcohol used as a sweetener. It's a member of the polyol family.

marinate   To soak meat, seafood, or other food in a seasoned sauce, called a marinade, which has a high acid content. The acids break down the muscle of the meat, making it tender and adding flavor.

menu planning   A plan of what you intend to prepare and serve for meals for a duration of time such as a week or month.

millet   A small seed. Find it in health food stores, often in the bulk grain area.

molasses   A thick syrup produced from sugars. It's a source of fructose.

molecule   The smallest particle of a substance that retains its chemical and physical properties.

monounsaturated fats   The most heart-friendly fat. Olive and canola oil are examples of monounsaturated fats.

motility disorder   A disorder that contributes to abnormal intestinal contractions.

mindful eating   A practice of eating in which you give your full attention to the eating process.

Neufchâtel cheese   A soft, unripened cheese originating from France.

oat flour   Whole oats that have been ground to a flour.

oligosaccharides   Carbohydrates that contain a relatively small number of chains of sugar.

olive oil   A fragrant liquid produced by crushing or pressing olives. Extra-virgin olive oil is the oil produced from the first pressing of a batch of olives; oil is also produced from other pressings after the first. Extra-virgin olive oil is generally considered the most flavorful and highest quality and is the type you want to use when your focus is on the oil itself.

omega-3 fatty acids   The fats associated with lowering the risk of heart attack and stroke. They also play a role in heart health and brain function.

osmotic diarrhea   Diarrhea that occurs when excess water is drawn into the intestine, often when foods are malasorped.

orzo   A rice-shape pasta.

paprika   A red-colored spice made from dried peppers.

Parmesan   A hard, dry, flavorful cheese primarily used grated or shredded as a seasoning for Italian-style dishes.

parsley   A fresh-tasting green leafy herb used to add color and interest to just about any savory dish. It's often used as a garnish just before serving.

peanut oil   A pale yellow oil with a nutty flavor. Peanut oil has a high smoking point, which means it can be heated to high temperatures without smoking.

penne   A short, tubelike pasta with diagonal-cut ends. In Latin, *penne* means "feather" or "quill."

phytochemicals   Plant substances linked with decreasing the risk for certain diseases.

pine nuts (also **pignoli** or **piñon**)   Nuts grown on pine trees that are rich (read: high fat), flavorful, and a bit pine-y. Pine nuts are a traditional component of pesto and add a wonderful hearty crunch to many other recipes.

pita bread   A flat, hollow wheat bread that can be used for sandwiches or cut, pizza style, into slices. Pita bread is terrific soft with dips or baked or broiled as a vehicle for other ingredients.

polenta   A cornmeal porridge that's a popular alternative to pasta or rice in Northern Italy. Find precooked polenta in some large grocery stores in the international section. Look for it in a tubelike shape, precooked and ready to slice to cook.

polyols   Substances that chemically resemble both sugars and alcohols and are often referred as sugar alcohols. Used often in sugar-free gum and mints as sweeteners, polyols can contribute to osmotic diarrhea.

polysaccharides   Complex chains of sugar molecules.

polyunsaturated fats   Fats that contain more than one double bond. Typically, polyunsaturated fats are liquid at room temperature.

portion size   The size of appropriate amount of food to eat at a meal or snack time based on your calorie needs.

portobello mushroom   A grown-up crimini mushroom that's low in fat and rich in fiber.

prebiotics   The undigested food that provides nourishment for the probiotics residing in your large intestine.

preheat   To turn on an oven, broiler, or other cooking appliance in advance of cooking so the temperature will be at the desired level when the assembled dish is ready for cooking.

probiotics   Live microorganisms that may include bacteria that provide your body positive health benefits.

prosciutto   A specialty ham from Italy that's air-cured.

quinoa   A South American grain rich in protein.

resveratrol   A powerful antioxidant that's been shown in studies to possibly lower risk of obesity and diabetes. Some research suggests that resveratrol may also have anti-inflammatory effects.

rice flour   A wheat-free and gluten-free flour. Look for it in health food stores or possibly in the gluten-free section of your grocery store.

rice milk   A grain milk made from rice that is lactose-free and tends to be far lower in protein than cow's milk.

rice pasta   A pasta very similar to traditional wheat pasta. Find it in health food stores or in the gluten-free sections of some grocery stores.

risotto   A popular Italian rice dish made by browning arborio rice in butter or oil and then slowly adding liquid to cook the rice. The result is a creamy-textured rice.

sage   An herb with a musty yet fruity, lemon-rind scent and "sunny" flavor. It's a terrific addition to many dishes.

satay   A popular southeast Asian dish made of marinated meat and served on skewers.

saturated fats   Fats that are generally solid at room temperature and linked to heart disease and stroke. Animal fats are typically rich in saturated fats.

sauté   To pan-cook over lower heat than used for frying.

serotonin   A hormone manufactured in the brain and gut. Ninety-five percent of the body's serotonin is in the intestines. People with IBS tend to have abnormal amounts of serotonin in their gastrointestinal tract. This elevated serotonin level impacts bowel motility, movements, and pain sensations.

serving size   The portion of food that's used as a reference on a nutrition facts label.

sesame oil   An oil that infuses a nutty flavor reminiscent of many Asian dishes. Sesame oil may lower blood pressure, is a good source of heart-healthy monounsaturated fats, and is rich in disease-fighting antioxidants. Find it in the Asian or international section of most grocery stores.

shred   To cut into many long, thin slices.

simmer   To boil gently so the liquid barely bubbles.

skewers   Thin wooden or metal sticks, usually about 8 inches long, used to assemble kebabs, dip food pieces into hot sauces, or serve single-bite food items with a bit of panache.

skillet (also **frying pan**)   A generally heavy, flat-bottomed metal pan with a handle designed to cook food over heat on a stovetop or campfire.

slice   To cut into thin pieces.

small intestinal bacterial overgrowth   When the small bowel is overrun with bacteria not normally found there.

soluble fiber   Fiber that mixes with water and forms a gel in the body. Studies suggest soluble fiber is best tolerated in IBS.

soy milk   A nondairy milk product made from soybeans and water.

steam   To suspend a food over boiling water and allow the heat of the steam (water vapor) to cook the food. Steaming is a very quick cooking method that preserves the flavor and texture of a food.

steel-cut oats   A very hearty form of oatmeal high in fiber and protein. Steel-cut oats are whole-grain oats taken from the inner part of the oat kernel.

stock   A flavorful broth made by cooking meats or vegetables with seasonings until the liquid absorbs these flavors. This liquid is then strained and the solids discarded. Stock can be eaten by itself or used as a base for soups, stews, sauces, risotto, or many other recipes.

stratas   A flavorful bread-and-egg pudding dish.

tahini   A sesame seed paste similar in consistency to natural peanut butter. Look for tahini at most grocery stores with the peanut butter or in the Middle Eastern section.

tandoori   A yogurt marinade popular in Indian cooking.

thyroid dysfunction   A disorder caused by an under- or overactive thyroid gland.

trans fats   Dietary fats associated with an increased risk of heart disease and stroke. Trans fats are created when liquid oils are changed to a more solid form in the process called hydrogenation.

turmeric   A bright yellow spice often used in Indian cooking. Studies have suggested that the chemical curcumin, found in turmeric, may have anti-inflammatory and anti-cancer properties.

visceral hypersensitivity   An increased sensitivity to pain and bloating often experienced by people with IBS.

walnuts   A nut with a rich, slightly woody flavor. They are delicious toasted and make fine accompaniments to cheeses.

water chestnuts   Actually a tuber, water chestnuts are a popular element in many types of Asian-style cooking. The flesh is white, crunchy, and juicy, and the vegetable holds its texture whether cool or hot.

whisk   To rapidly mix, introducing air to the mixture.

whole-wheat flour   Wheat flour that contains the entire grain.

xylitol   A sugar alcohol used as a sweetener. It's a member of the polyol family.

zest   Small slivers of peel, usually from a citrus fruit such as lemon, lime, or orange.

Appendix B

Resources

Now that you're on your journey to managing your IBS, you may want to learn more on some subjects that pertain specifically to *your* symptoms. Unfortunately, there's lots of misinformation out there, so knowing where to find the legitimate sources is important. This appendix provides great books and websites to further your knowledge in IBS management. Check out the great cookbook selections, too!

IBS and Nutrition

Catsos, Patsy. *IBS-Free at Last*. Portland, ME: Pond Cove Press, 2008.

Joneja, Janice Vickerstaff. *Digestion, Diet and Disease: Irritable Bowel Syndrome and Gastrointestinal Function*. Rutgers, NJ: Rutgers University Press, 2004.

Lackner, Jeffrey. *Controlling IBS the Drug-Free Way*. New York, NY: Stewart, Tabori and Chang, 2007.

Magee, Elaine. *Tell Me What to Eat If I Have Irritable Bowel Syndrome*. Franklin Lakes, NJ: New Page Books, 2008.

National Institute of Diabetes and Digestive and Kidney Disease
www.niddk.nih.gov

The American College of Gastroenterology
acg.gi.org

Digestive Health

King, John. *Mayo Clinic on Digestive Health*. Rochester, MN: Mayo Clinic, 2004.

Lipski, Elisabeth. *Digestive Wellness*. New York, NY: McGraw-Hill, 2004.

Wheat-Free Diets and Celiac Disease

Case, Shelley. *Gluten-Free Diet*. Regina, Saskatchewan, Canada: Case Nutrition Consulting, 2008 (www.glutenfreediet.ca).

Celiac.com
www.celiac.com

Wheat-Free and Dairy-Free Cookbooks, Allergy Books, and More

Abraham, Ellen. *Simple Treats: A Wheat-Free, Dairy-Free Guide to Scrumptious Baked Goods*. Summertown, TN: Book Publishing Company, 2003.

Mallorca, Jacqueline. *The Wheat-Free Cook*. New York, NY: HarperCollins, 2007.

Melina, Vesanto, Jo Stepaniak, and Dina Aronson. *Food Allergy Survival Guide*. Summertown, TN: Healthy Living Publications, 2004.

The Food Allergy and Anaphylaxis Network
www.foodallergy.org

Living Without **Magazine**
www.livingwithout.com

Wheat-Free Product Companies

Arrowhead Mills
www.arrowheadmills.com

Bob's Red Mill Natural Foods, Inc.
www.bobsredmill.com

Blue Diamond Growers
www.bluediamond.com

Edward and Sons Trading Company, Inc.
www.edwardandsons.com

Food for Life Baking Company
www.foodforlife.com

Gluten-Free Pantry
www.glutenfreepantry.com

Nature's Path Foods
www.naturespath.com

Lactase Supplements, Probiotics, and Other Supplements

Lactase enzymes:

Lactaid McNeil Nutritionals
www.lactaid.com

Probiotics:

Align daily probiotic supplement
www.aligngi.com

Culturelle
www.culturelle.com

National Institutes of Health
National Center for Complementary and Alternative Medicine
nccam.nih.gov/health/probiotics

ConsumerLab.com
www.consumerlab.com

Index